Getting Ready for My Heart Cath

A Cardiac Catheterization Book for Kids – Preparation and Recovery

This book belongs to:

_____

Written by Dr. Fei Zheng-Ward　　　　Illustrated by Moch. Fajar Shobaru

Copyright © 2025 Fei Zheng-Ward

All rights reserved. Published by Fei Zheng-Ward, an imprint of FZWbooks. No part of this book may be copied, reproduced, recorded, transmitted, or stored by any means or in any form, electronic or mechanical, without obtaining prior written permission from the copyright owner.

Identifiers:　ISBN 979-8-89318-114-2 (eBook)
　　　　　　　ISBN 979-8-89318-115-9 (paperback)
　　　　　　　ISBN 979-8-89318-116-6 (hardcover)

Everyone is born with a heart, and some hearts are so special that they need a little extra love and care.

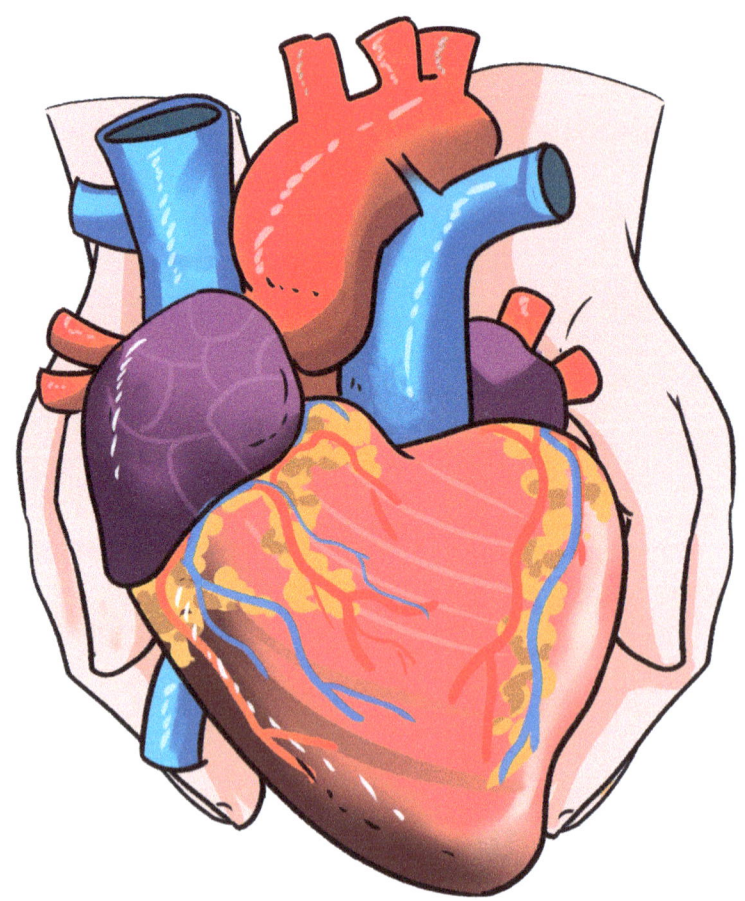

Do you have a special heart?

____ YES   ____ NO

Heart cath, also known as cardiac catheterization, is a test that your heart doctor performs to look at your special heart.

It checks things like (Check the ones that apply to you):

- ☐ How your heart valves are working
- ☐ The blood vessels that go in and out of your heart
- ☐ How blood flows in and out of your heart
- ☐ How much oxygen or pressure is in different parts of your heart and lungs
- ☐ How the different parts of your heart work together and "talk" to each other
- ☐ If you need surgery to repair your heart
- ☐ How your heart is doing after surgery

This test also lets your doctor:

- Close little "windows" between different parts of the heart
- Close blood vessels that are no longer needed
- Make small blood vessels or heart valve openings bigger
- Fix dancing heartbeats (arrhythmias)
- Take a tiny sample (biopsy) from the heart

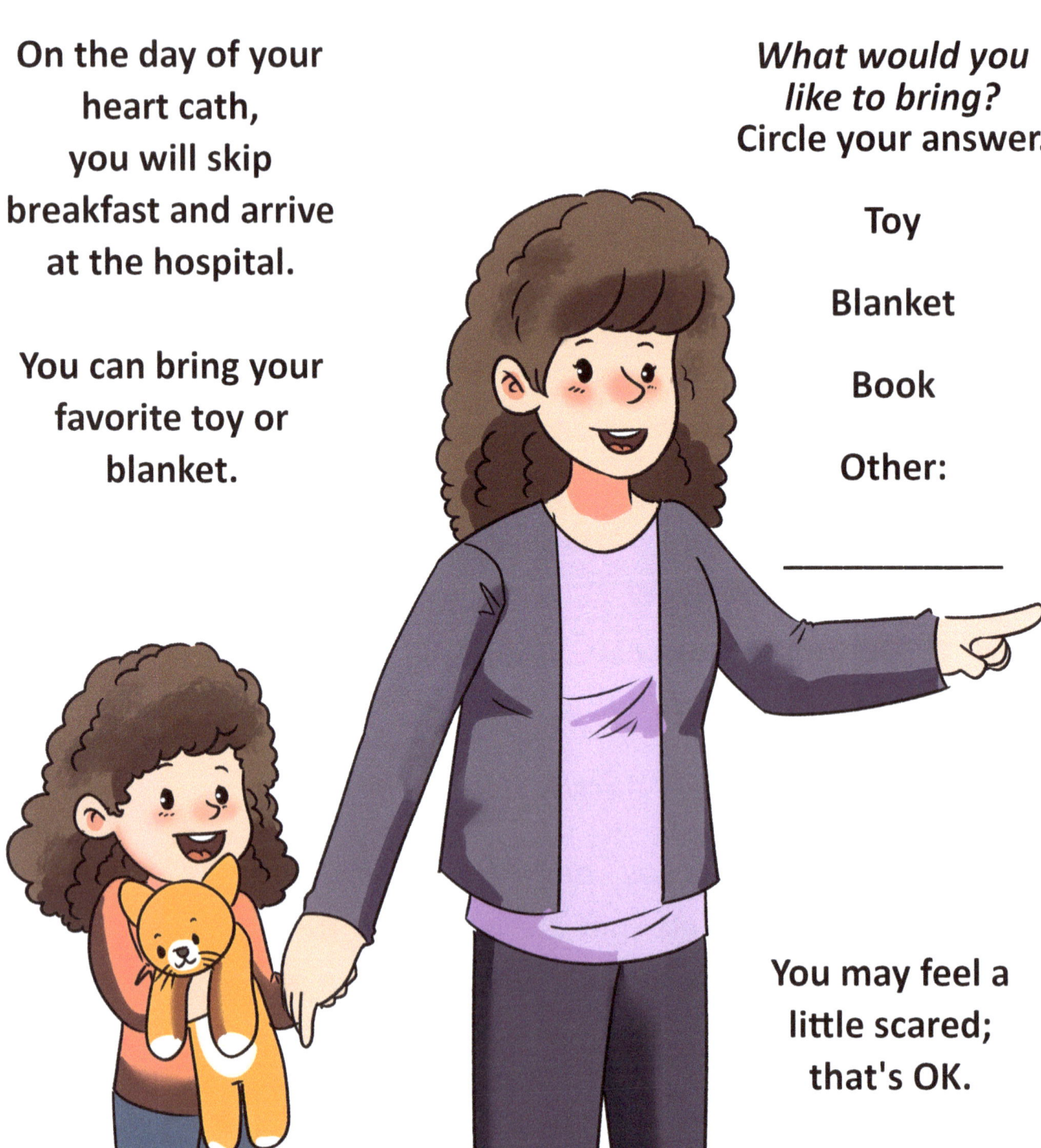

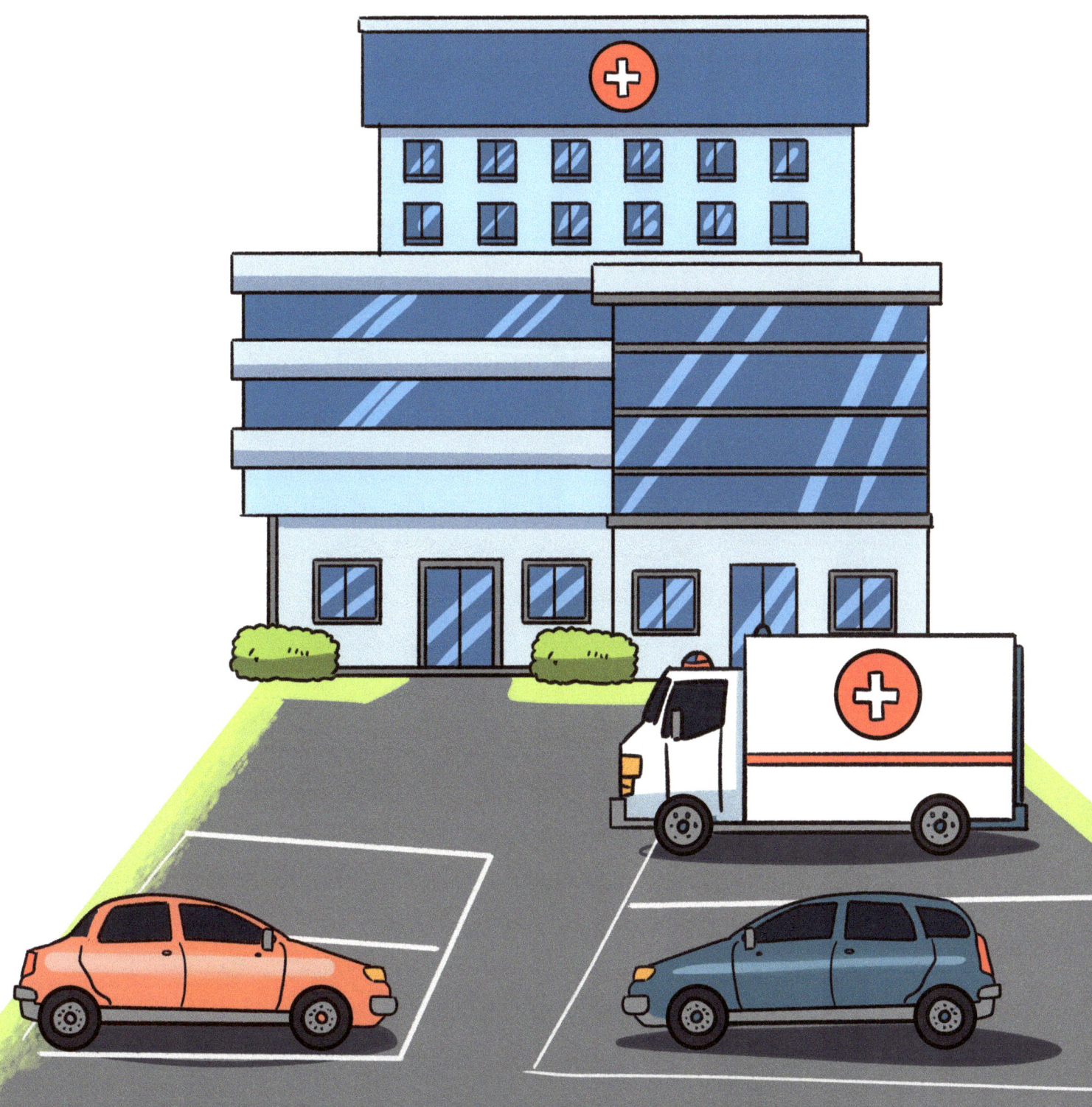

You will check in at the hospital and tell them your name and birthday.

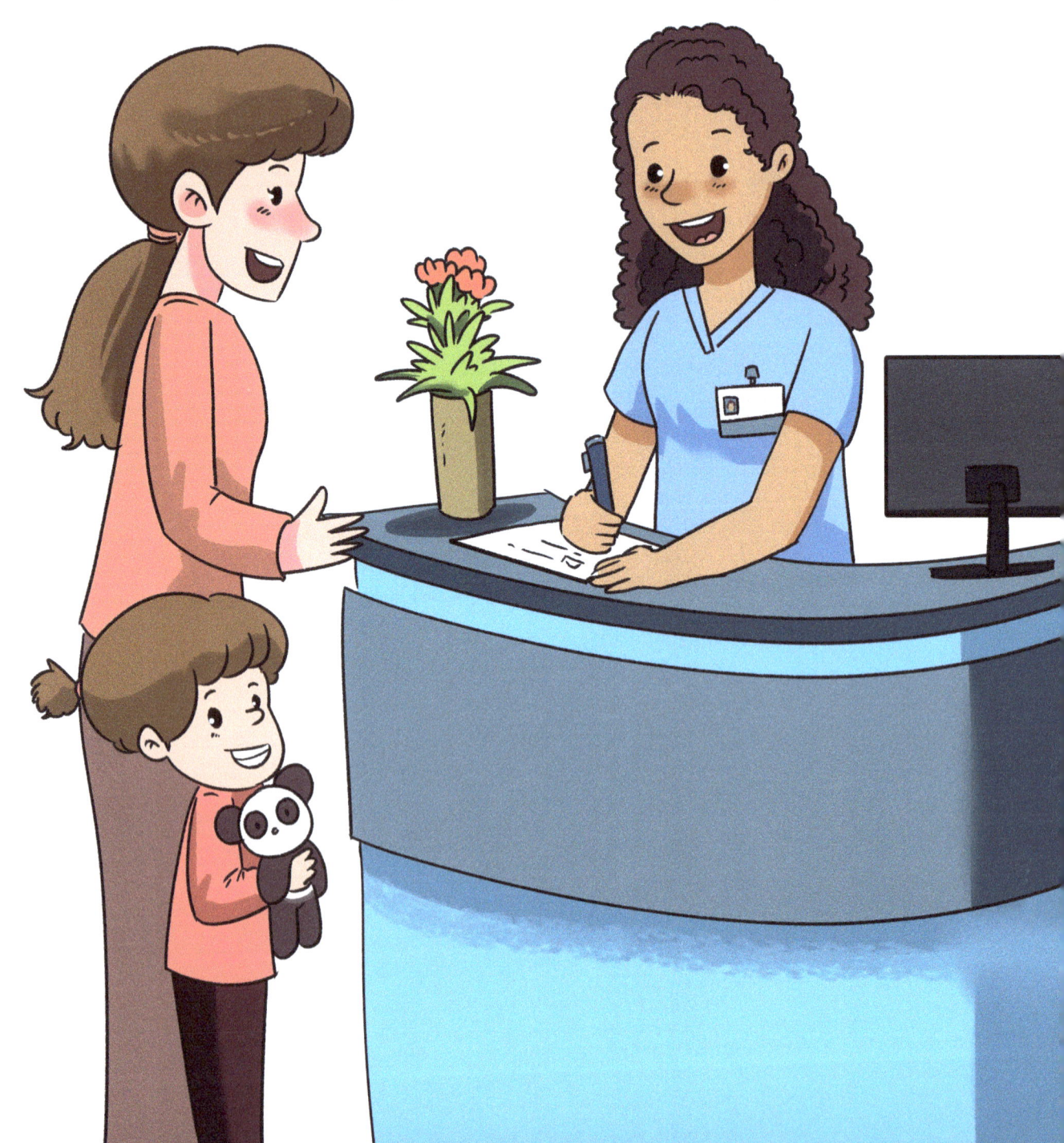

Then, you will get a special wristband.
Now everyone will know your name and birthday!

What color wristband will you get?
Circle the color of your wristband below.

Red   Green   Yellow   Blue   Pink   Orange

Purple   Black   White

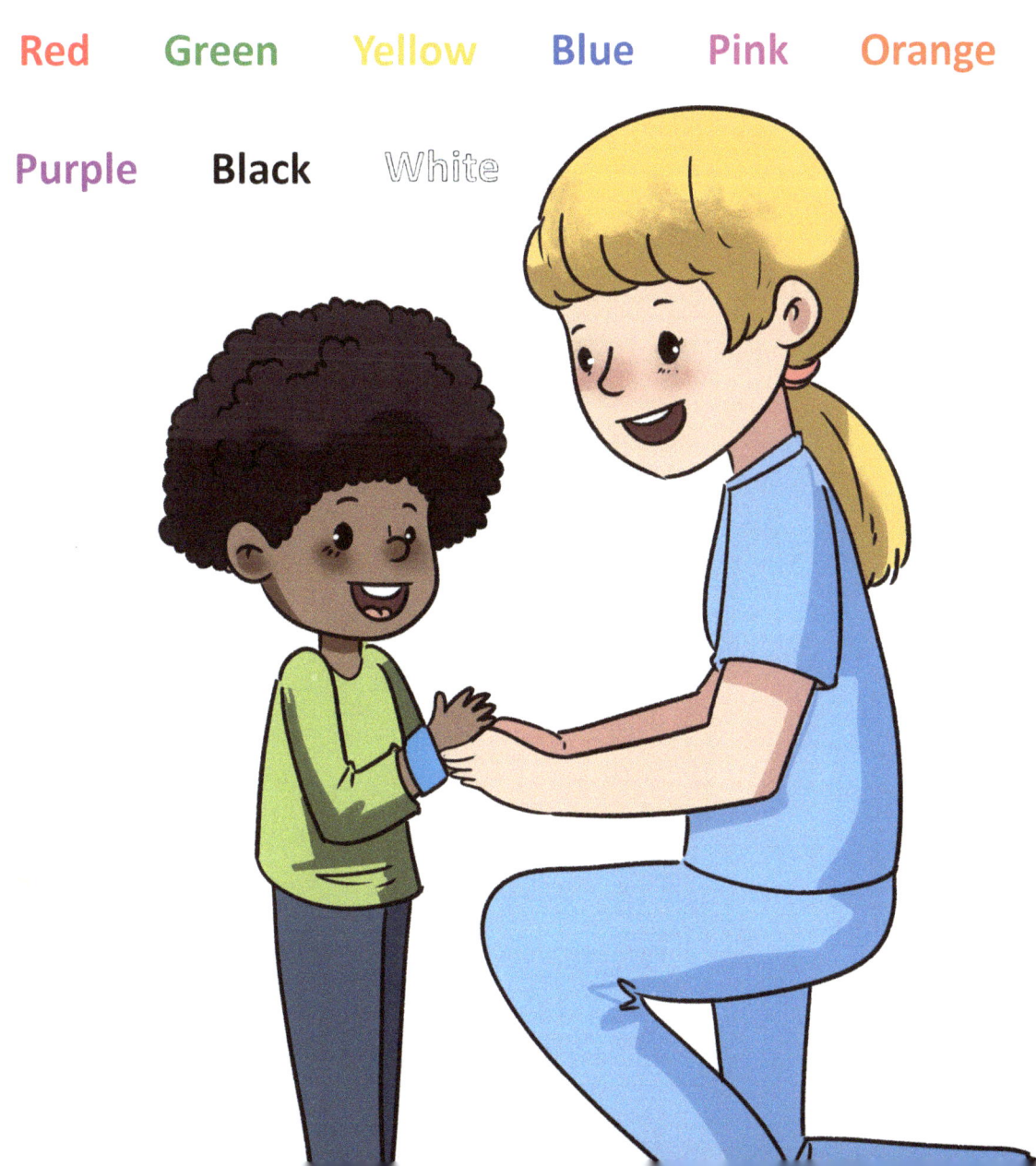

They will check your weight and height before getting you ready.

Do you know how much you weigh?

Do you know how tall you are?

My weight is:

_____

My height is:

_____

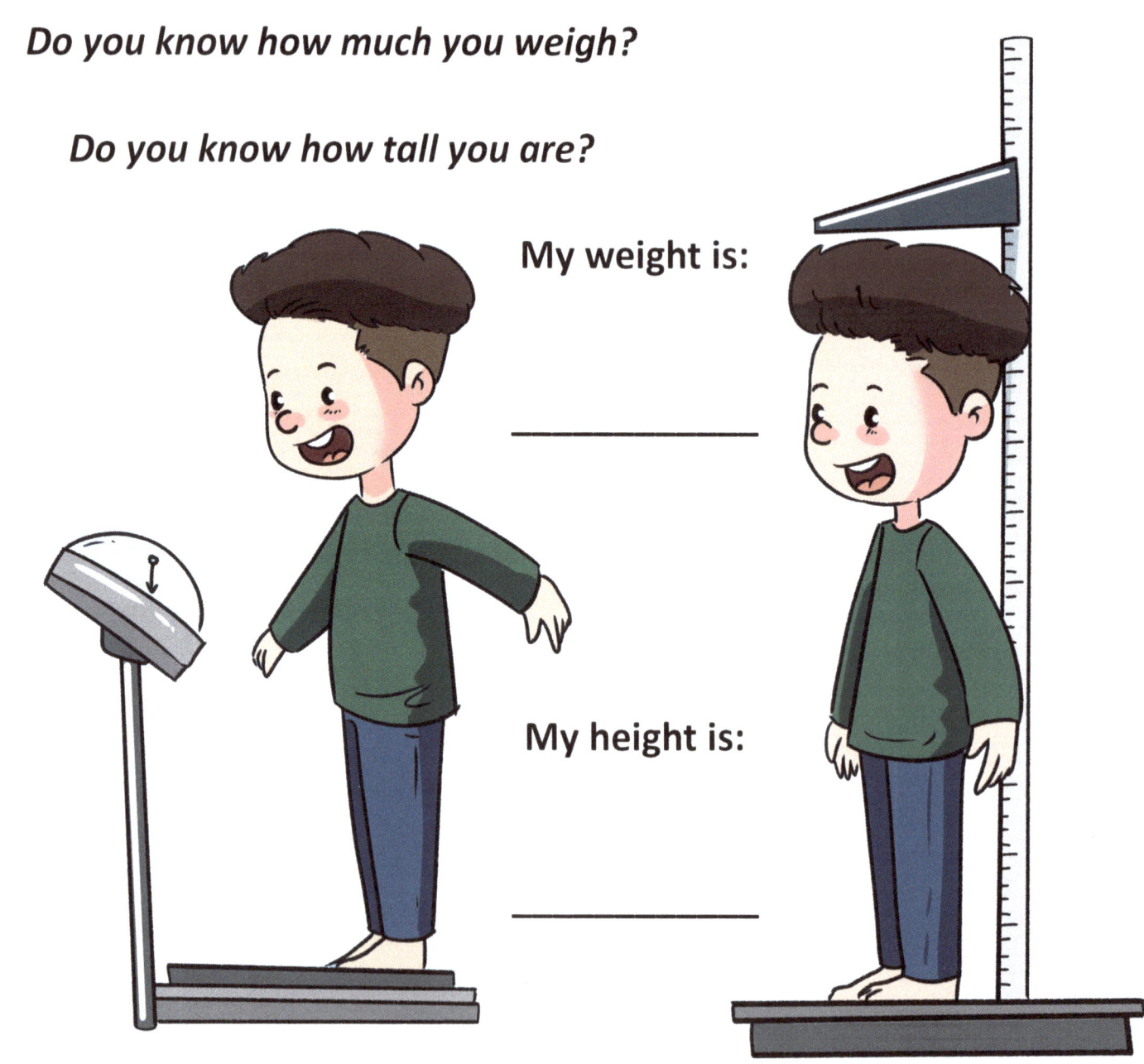

You will change into a new outfit, put on a hat, a gown (that looks like a backward superhero cape), and some cozy socks.

You've got this!

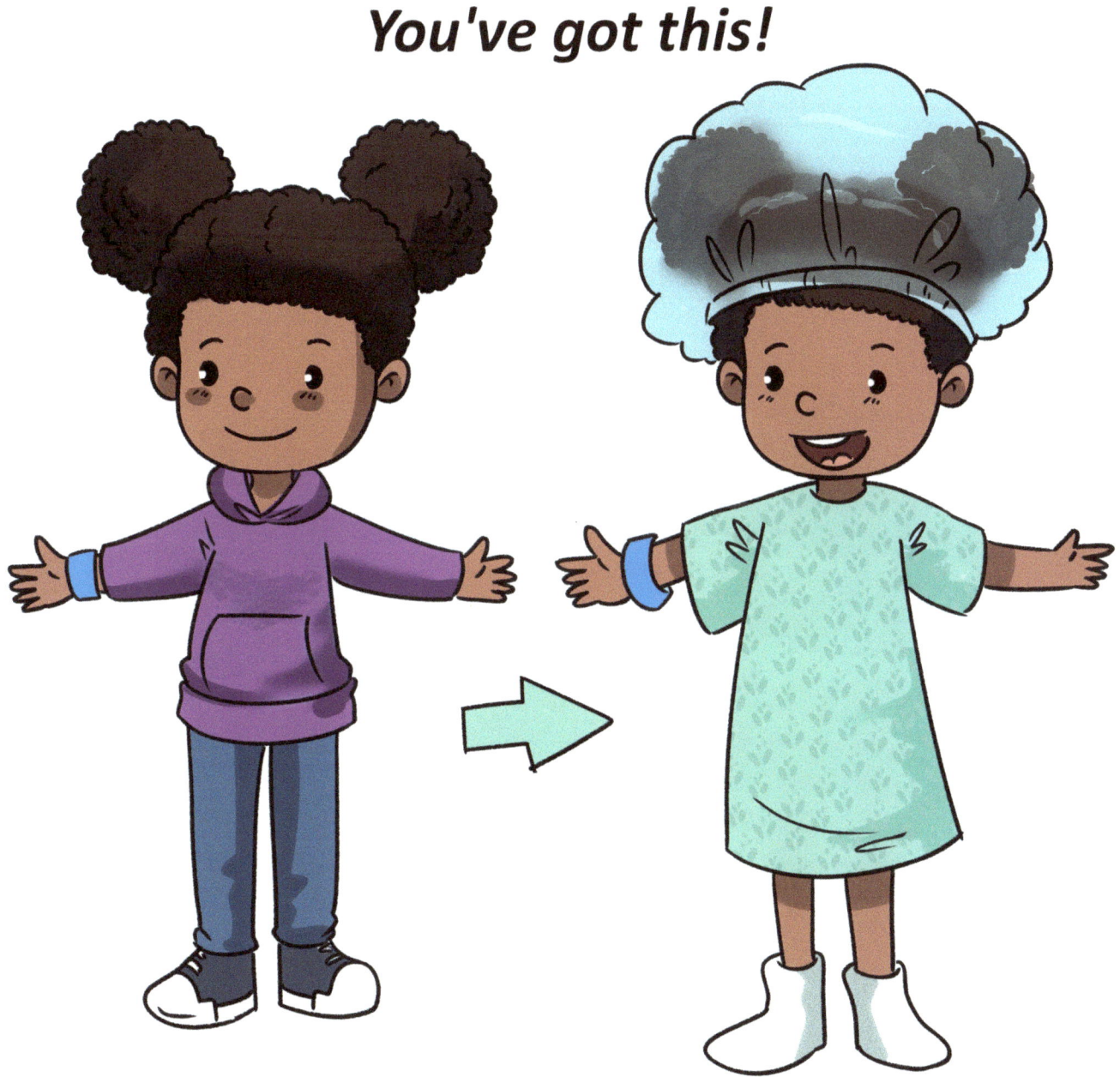

Your nurse will put a bandage-like tape or a clip on your finger or toe. It checks how much oxygen is in your body.

Oxygen helps your body work,
so you can do all the things you love!

What do you love to do?

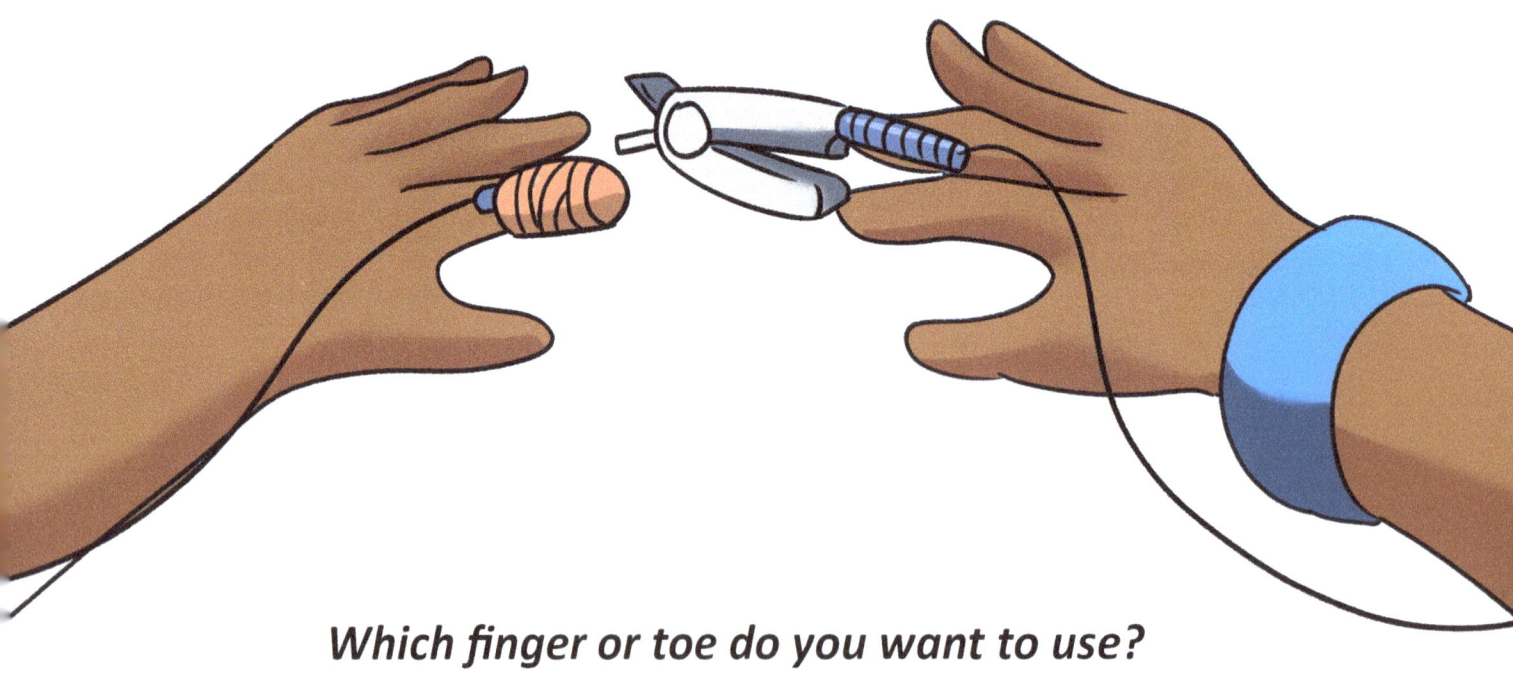

Which finger or toe do you want to use?

My vital signs are:

Temperature

_____

Blood Pressure

_____ / _____

Oxygen Level

_____ %

Heart Rate

_____ times per minute

Breathing

_____ times per minute

You'll get a blood pressure cuff around your arm or leg.
The cuff will give you a BIG squeeze.

Try your best to stay still.

Are you ready?

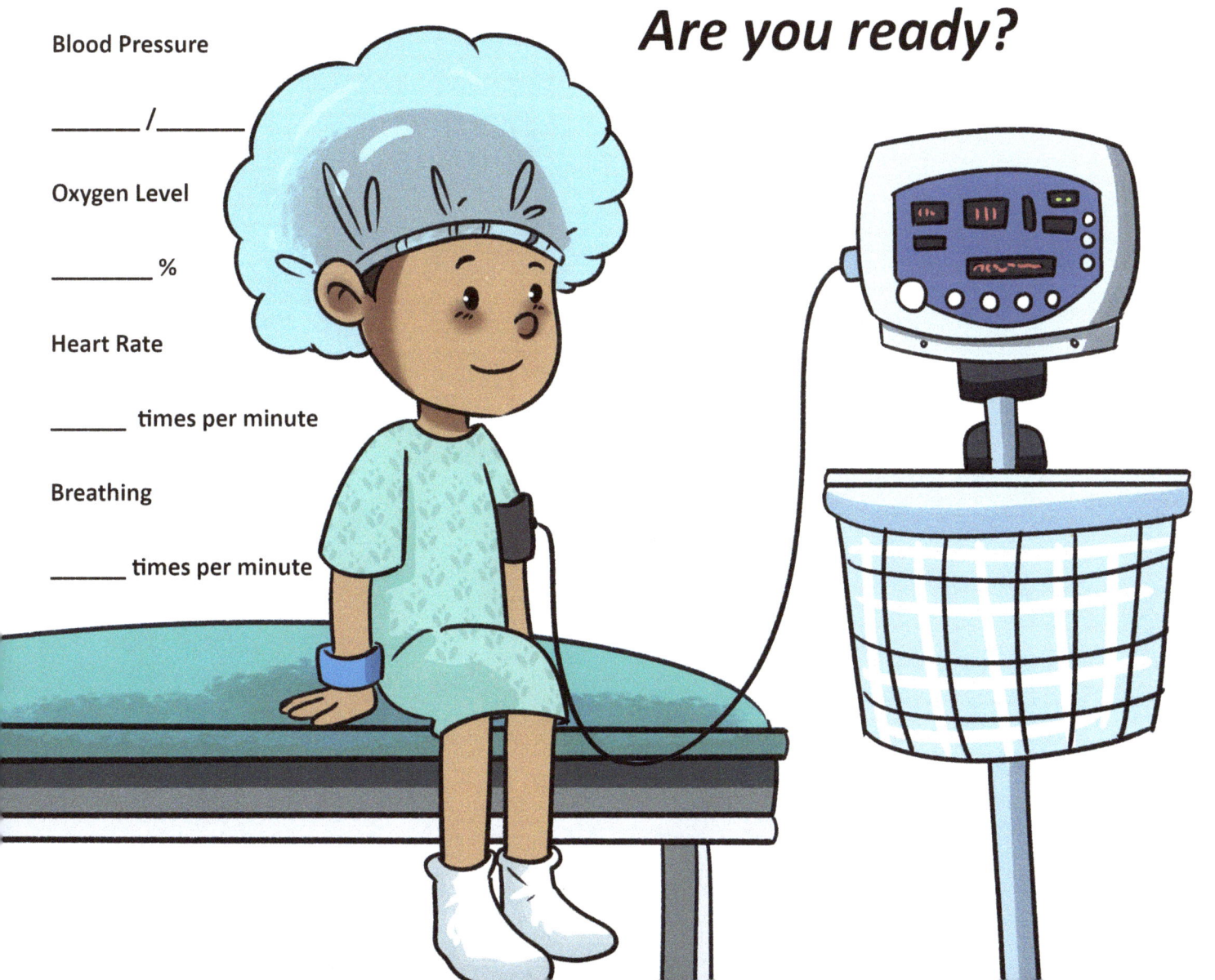

You and your parent or guardian will meet your heart and anesthesia doctors before your procedure.

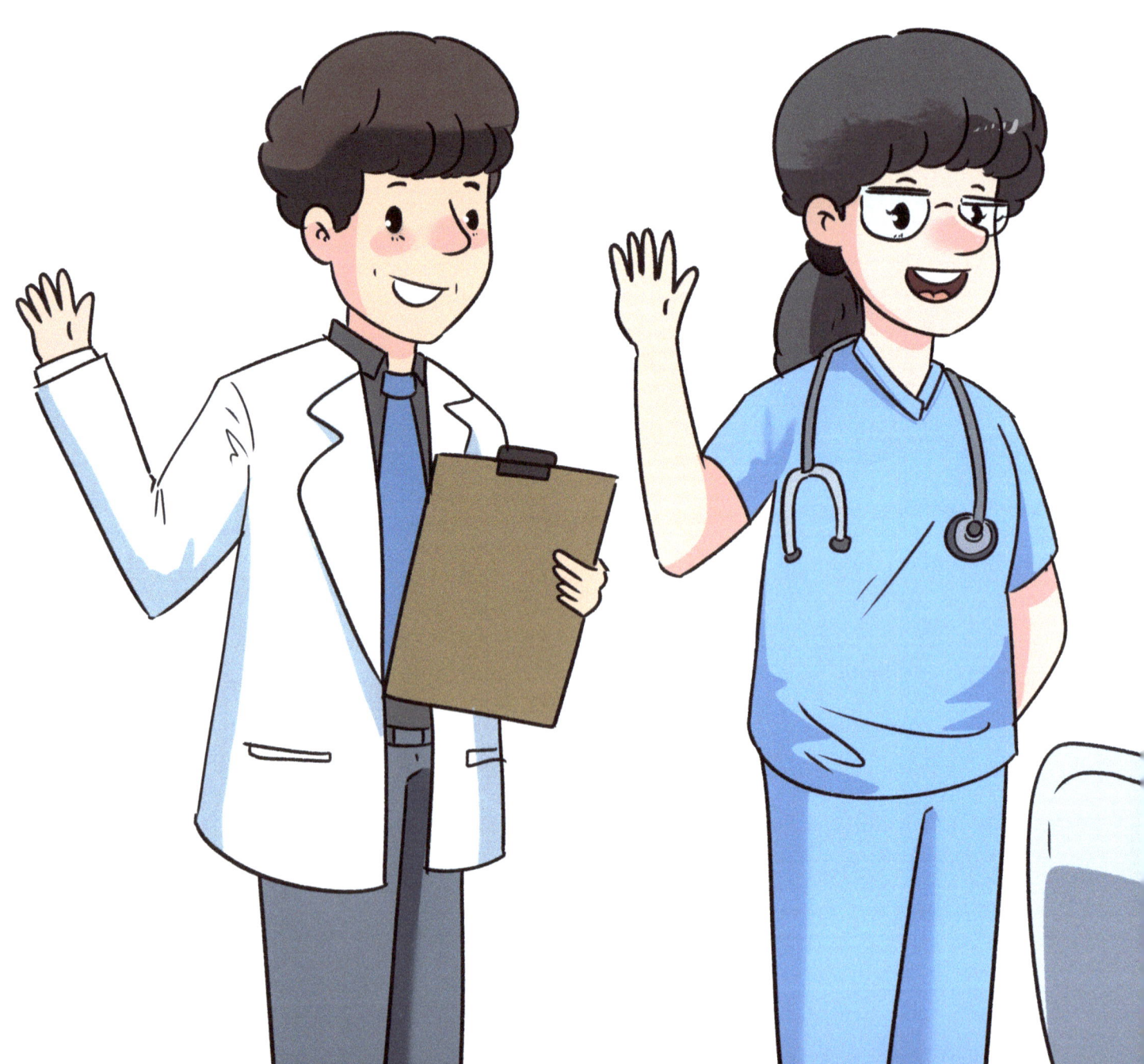

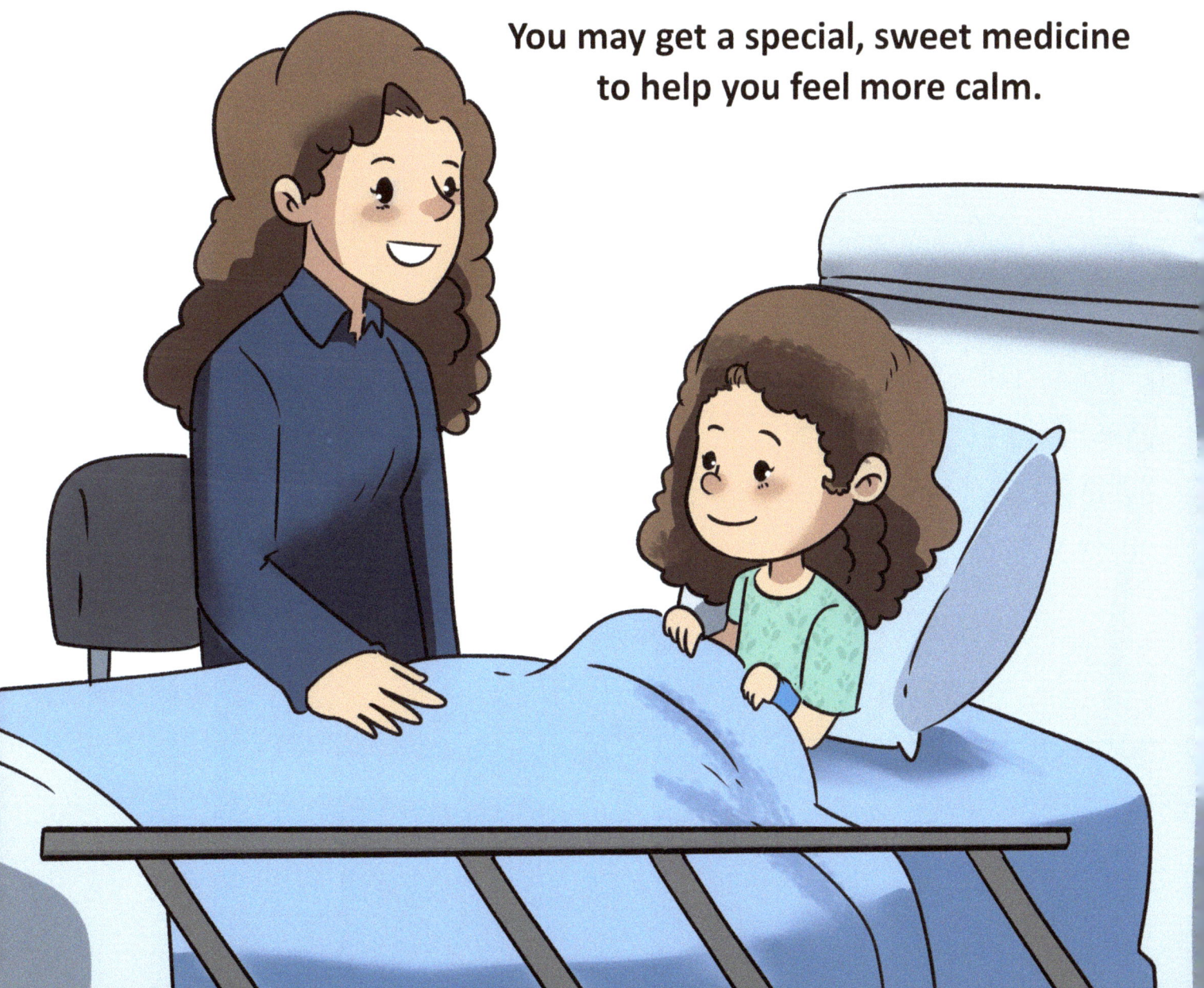

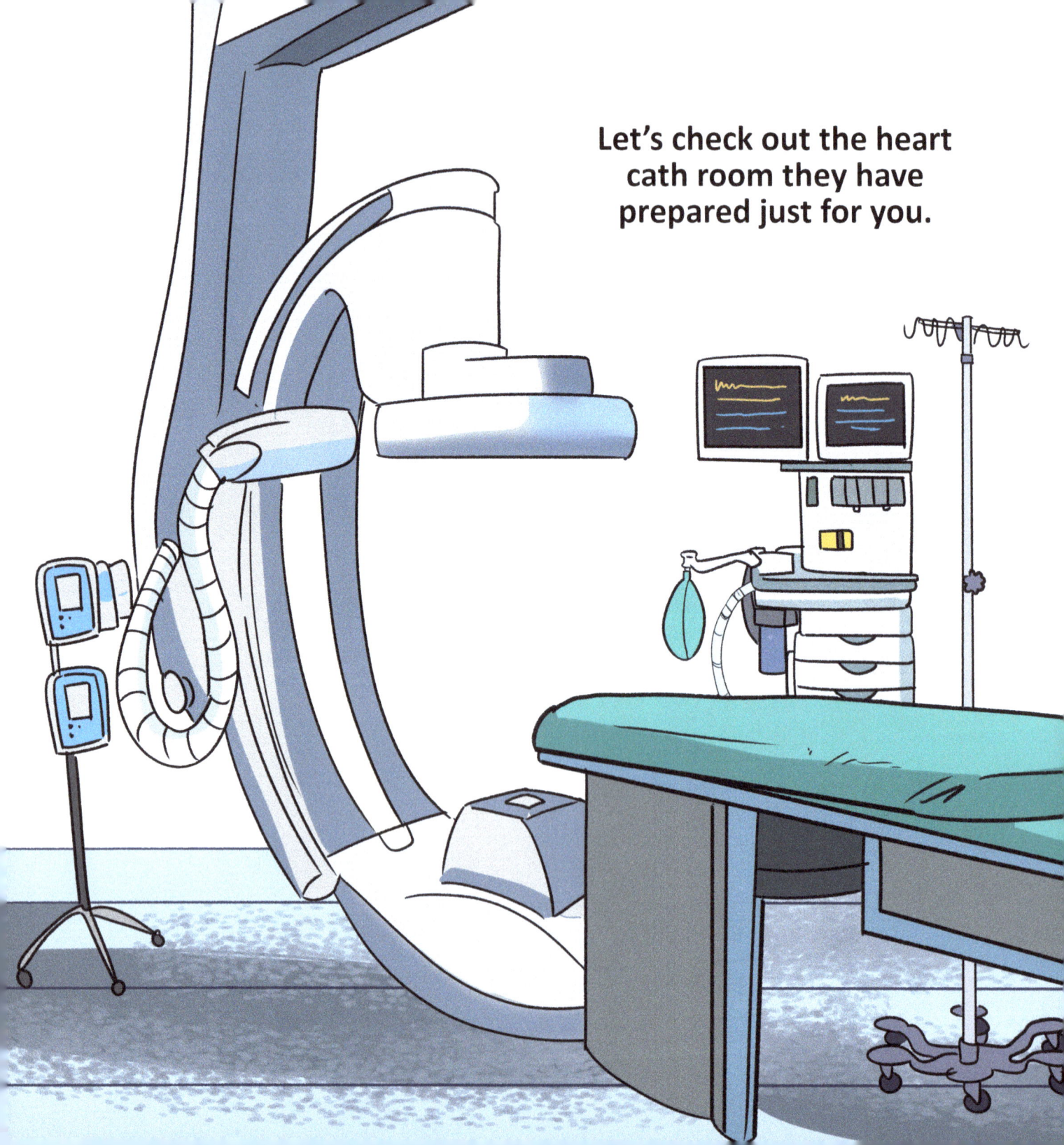

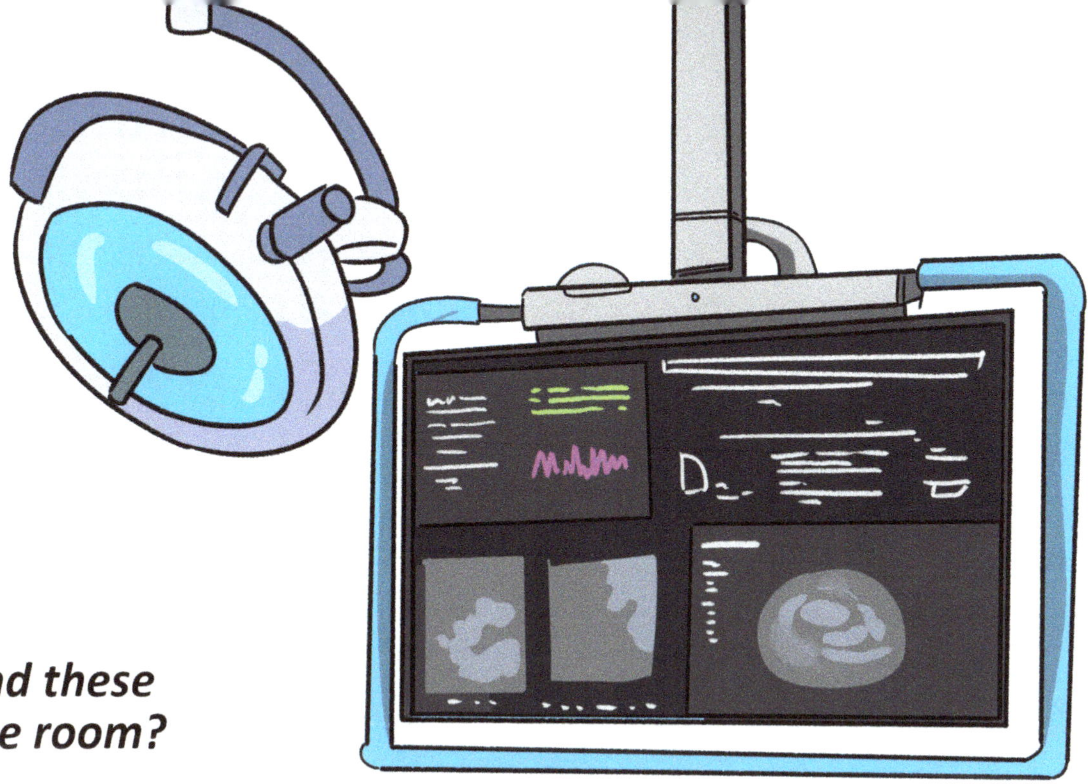

Can you find these things in the room?

- A bed in the middle of the room just for you
- A big C-shaped camera used to look at your heart
- A large computer monitor close to the bed
- A light hanging from the ceiling
- An IV (intravenous) pole for hanging bags of fluids and medicine
- An anesthesia machine with a balloon attached to it

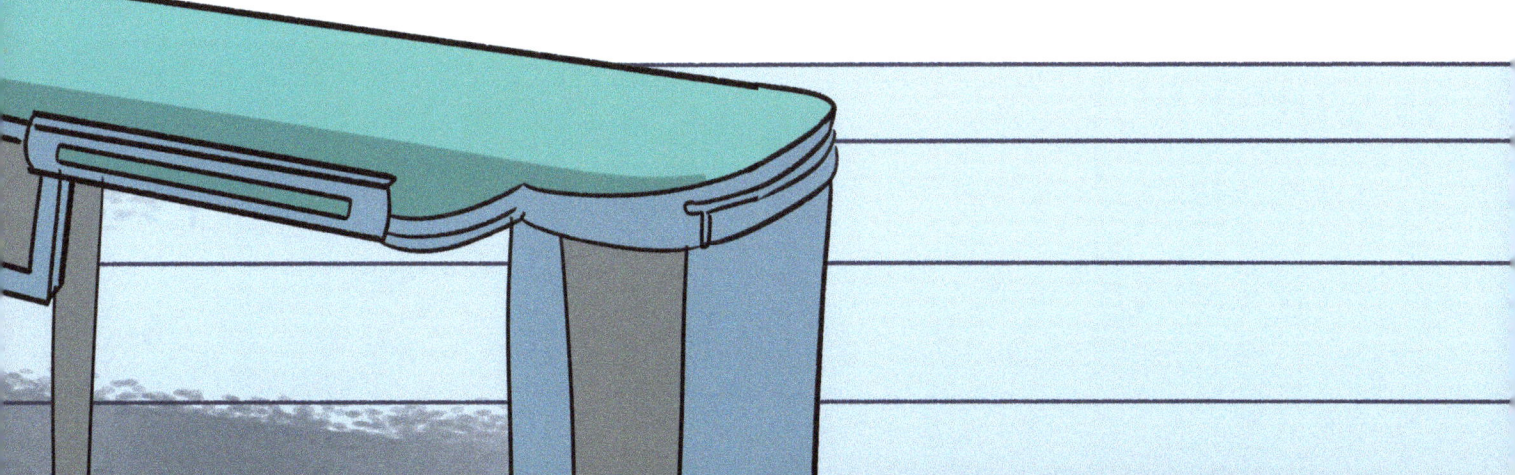

After you get on the bed in the middle of the room, they will check your heart, breathing, oxygen level, and blood pressure.

Small stickers called electrodes will be placed on your chest and arms to check your heart.

You can do this!

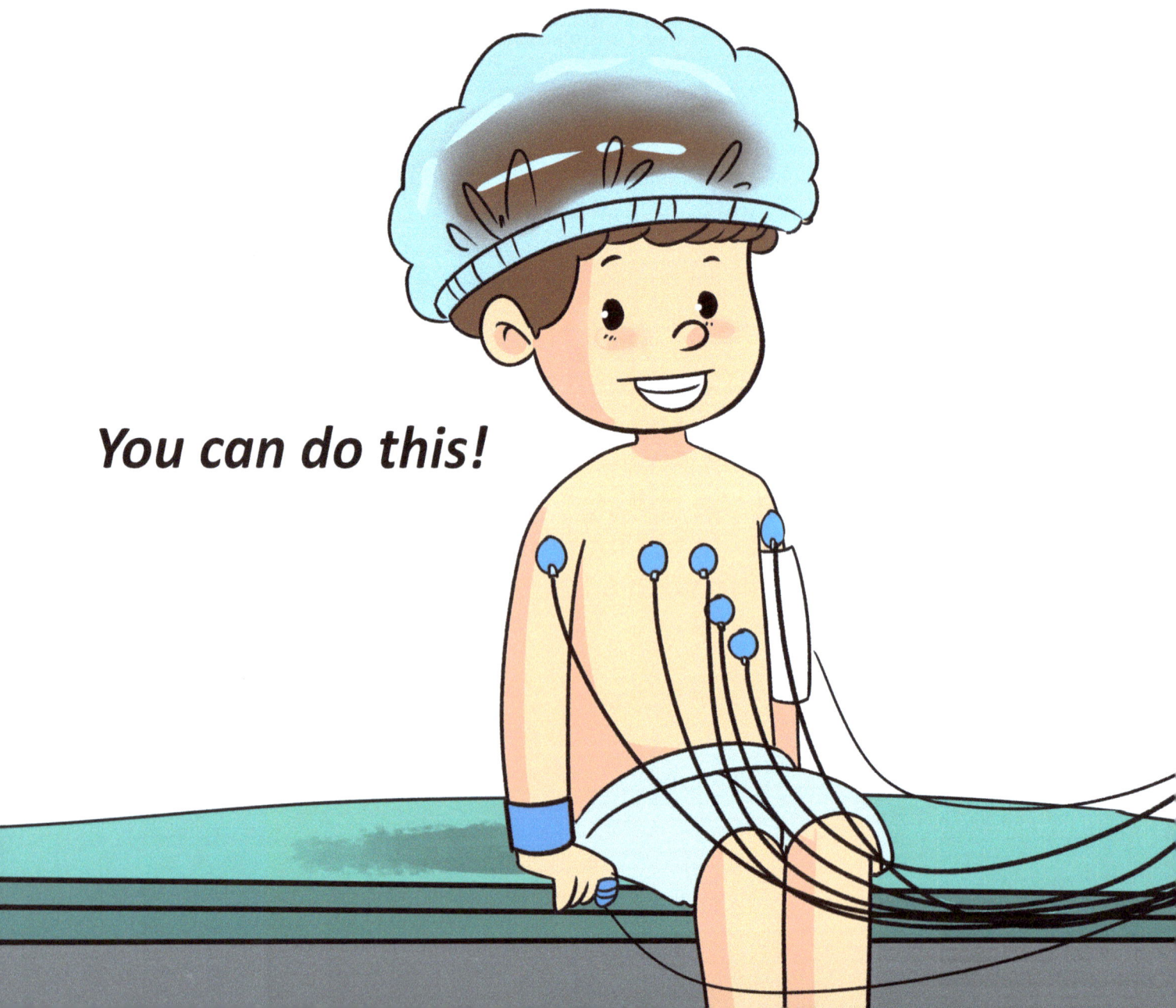

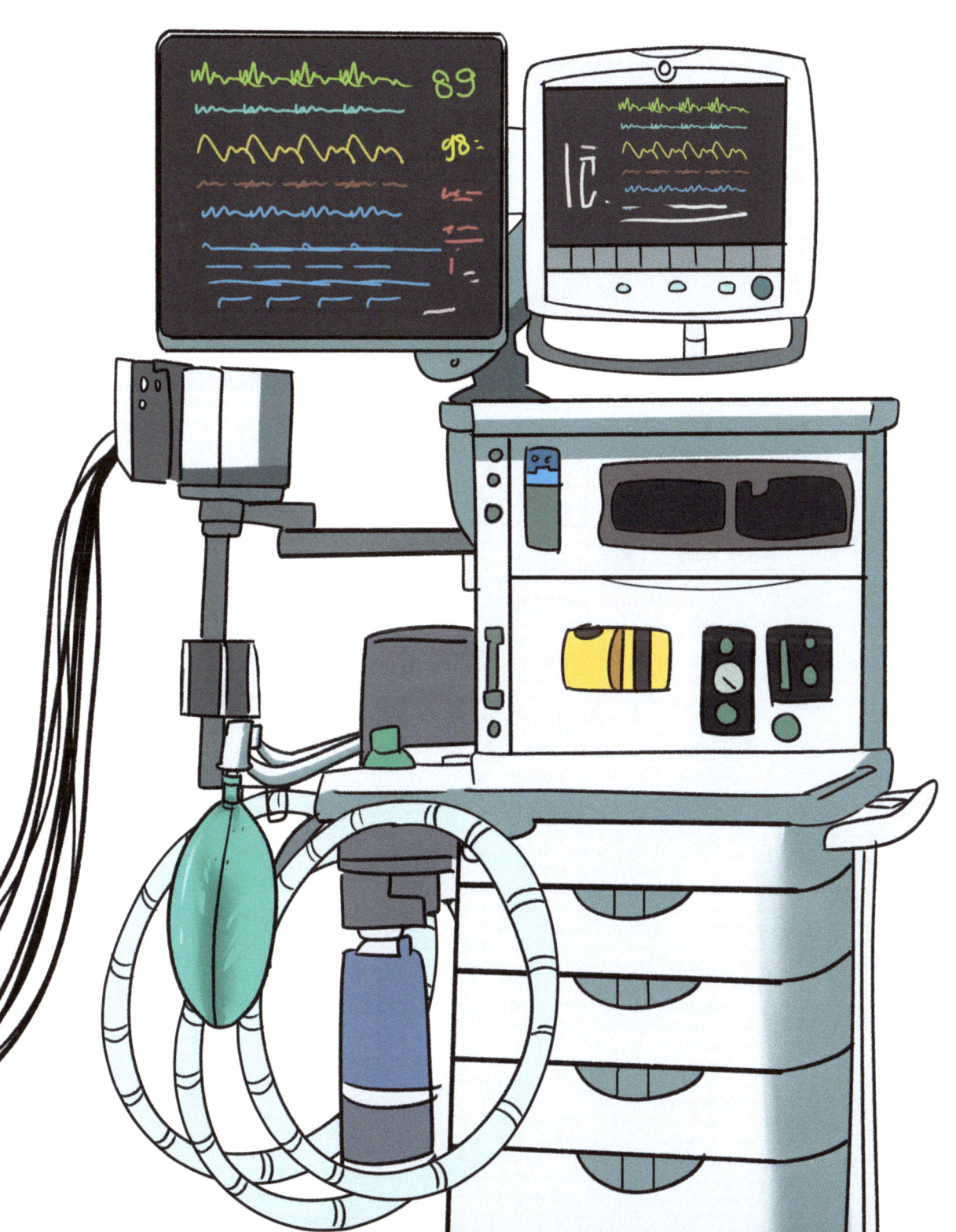

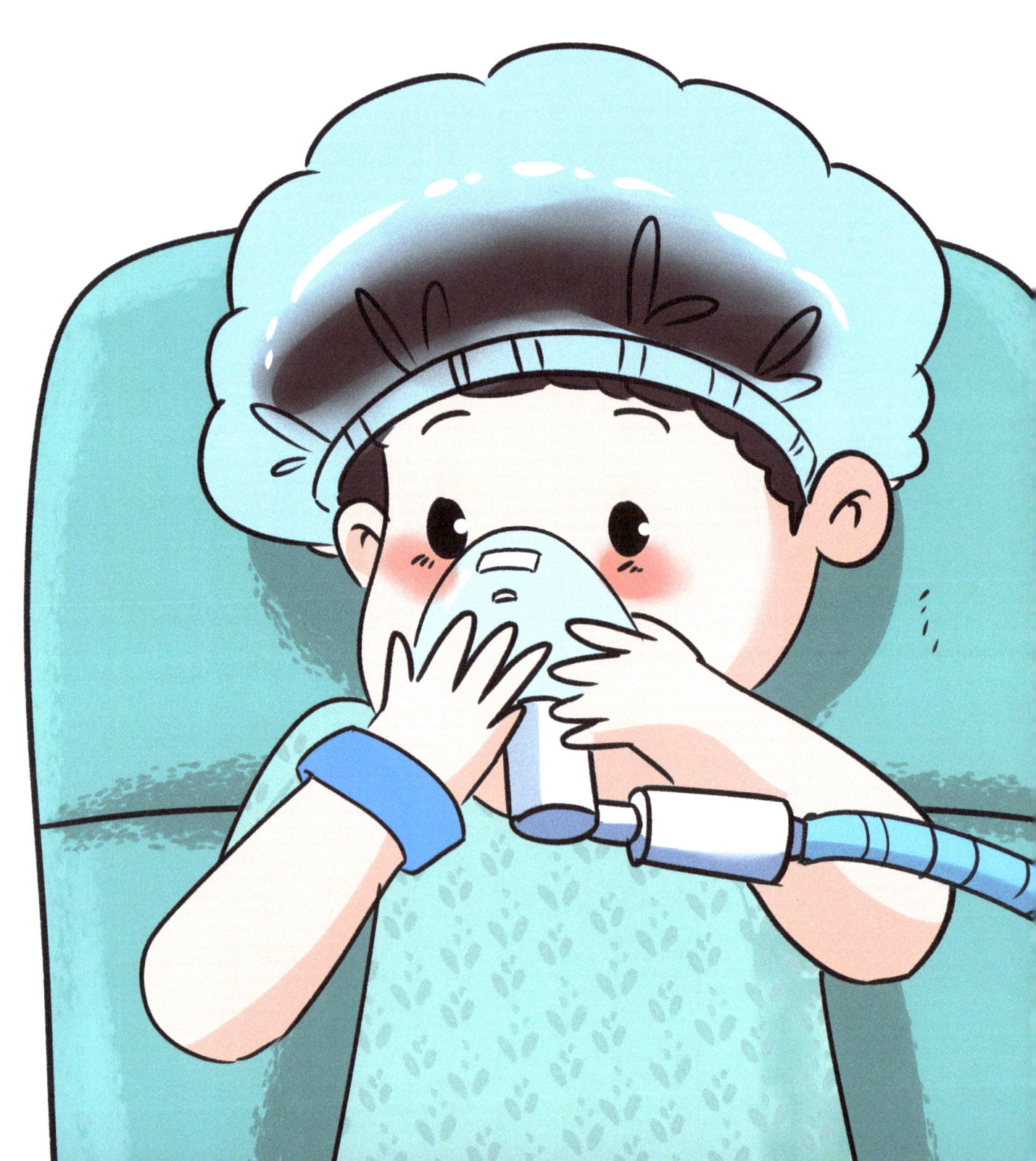

Your anesthesia doctor will give you a mask to breathe into.

Did you know they can make your mask smell sweet and yummy like bubble gum or your favorite fruit?

Draw or write down what scent you would like your mask to smell like:

_____

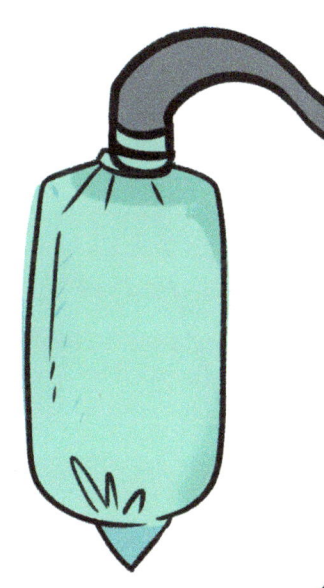

You can see your breathing by watching the balloon on the anesthesia machine.

Cool, right?

<u>Challenge</u>: *Can you blow into your mask and make the balloon bigger?*

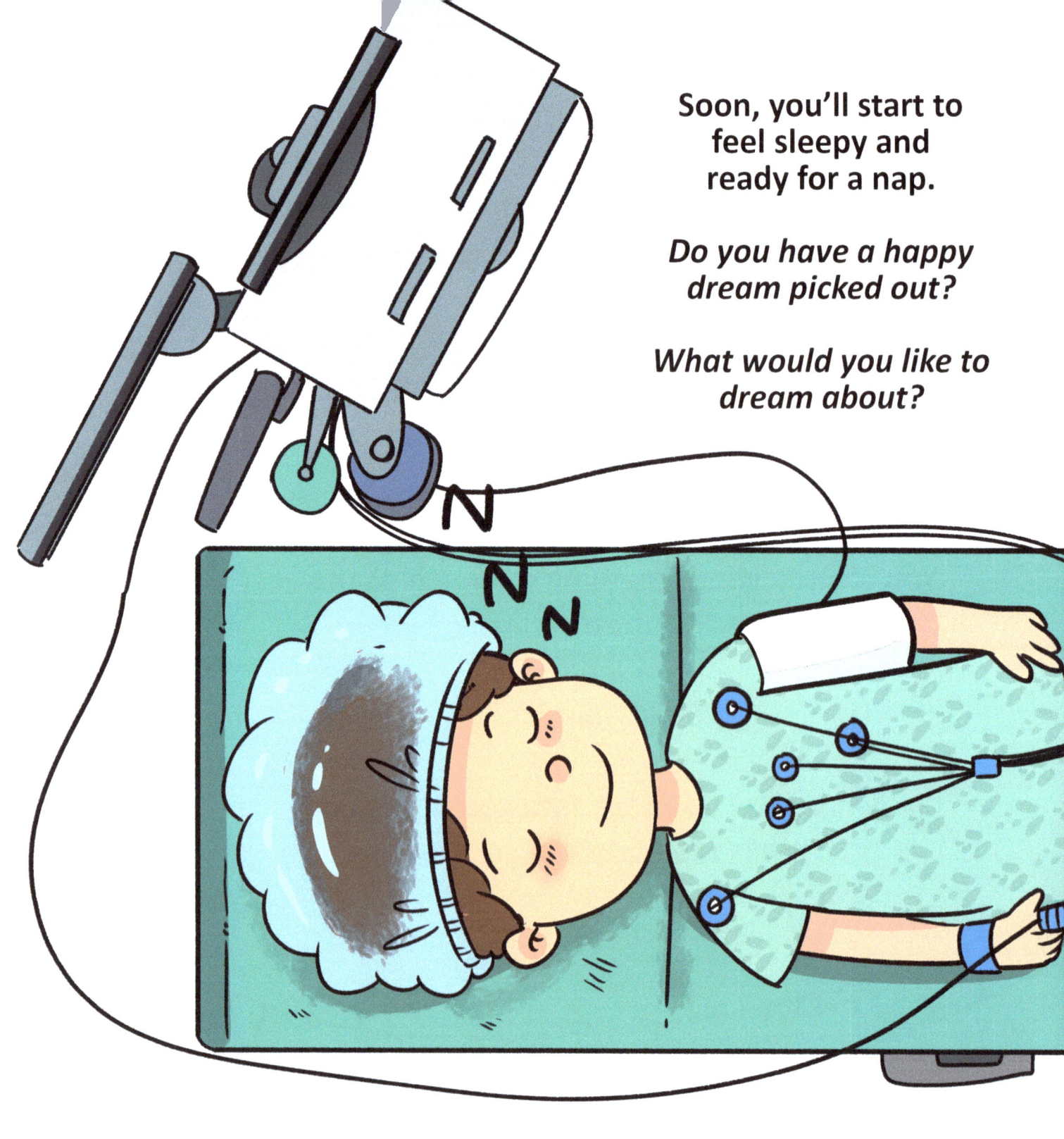

Your surgery will be done while you're dreaming away, and you won't feel a thing!

Your doctors and nurses will take good care of you and keep you safe and comfortable.

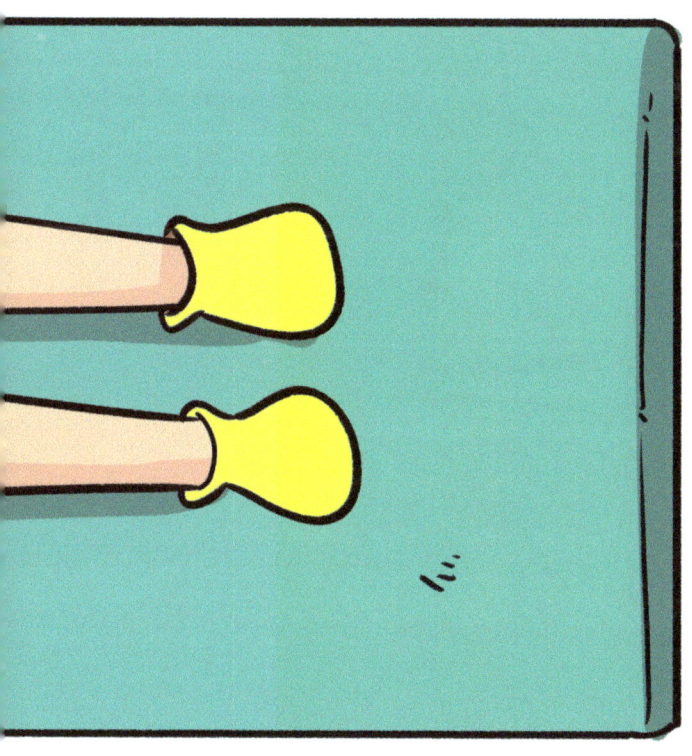

Sweet dreams...

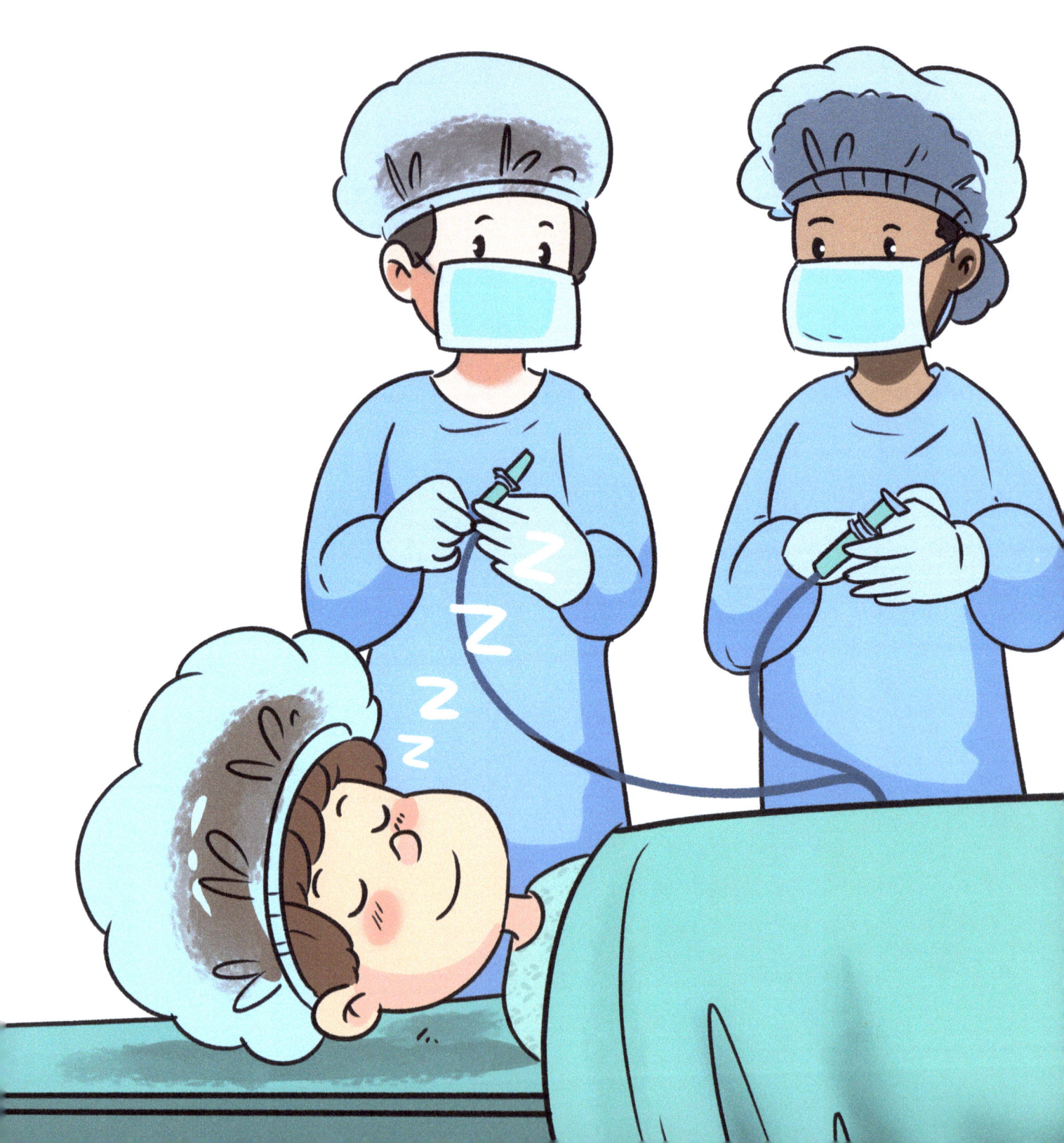

During the procedure, your doctor will gently and carefully put a long, skinny, bendable straw into a blood vessel in your groin, at the top of your leg.
Sometimes, they use your arm or neck instead of the groin.

This straw is like a tiny submarine that travels up your blood vessel to get to your heart. It helps the doctor see how to make your heart stronger and work better.

Sometimes, a special liquid medicine called contrast is used to help the doctor see different parts of your heart more clearly.

When the procedure is done, your doctor will remove the long, skinny straw, and you'll get a bandage on that spot.

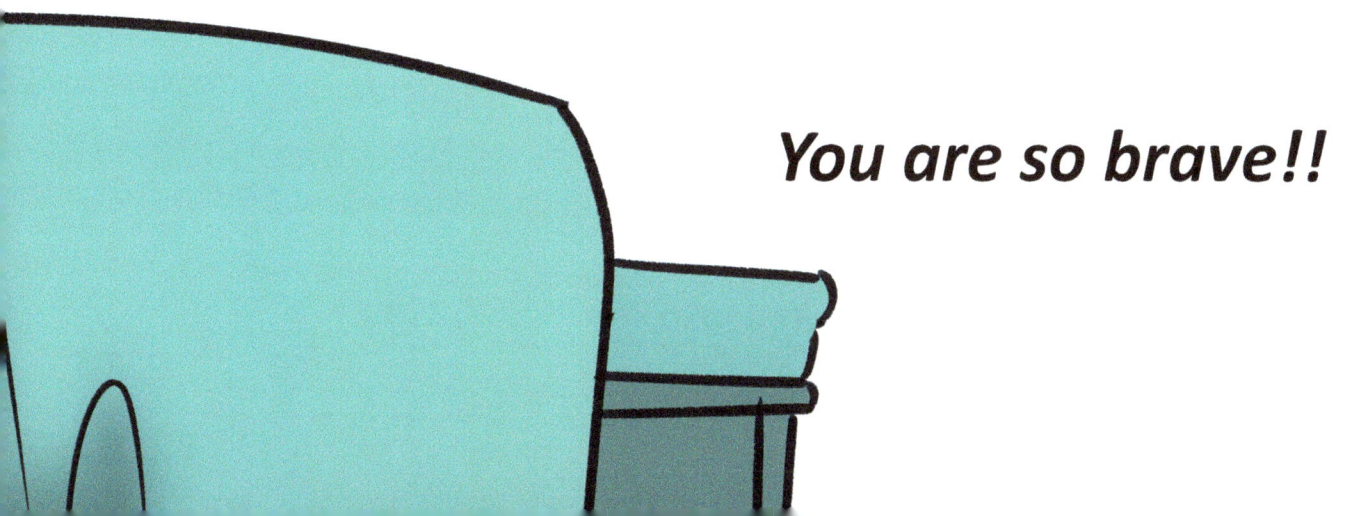

You are so brave!!

When you wake up from your nap, your procedure will be all done.

Your throat and groin may feel a little sore or uncomfortable.

If you need medicine to help you feel better, it will be given to you through the small plastic tube in your arm or leg. The tube was placed while you were sleeping.

Fun fact: The small plastic tubes, called IV catheters, come in fun colors like yellow, blue, pink, green, gray, and orange.

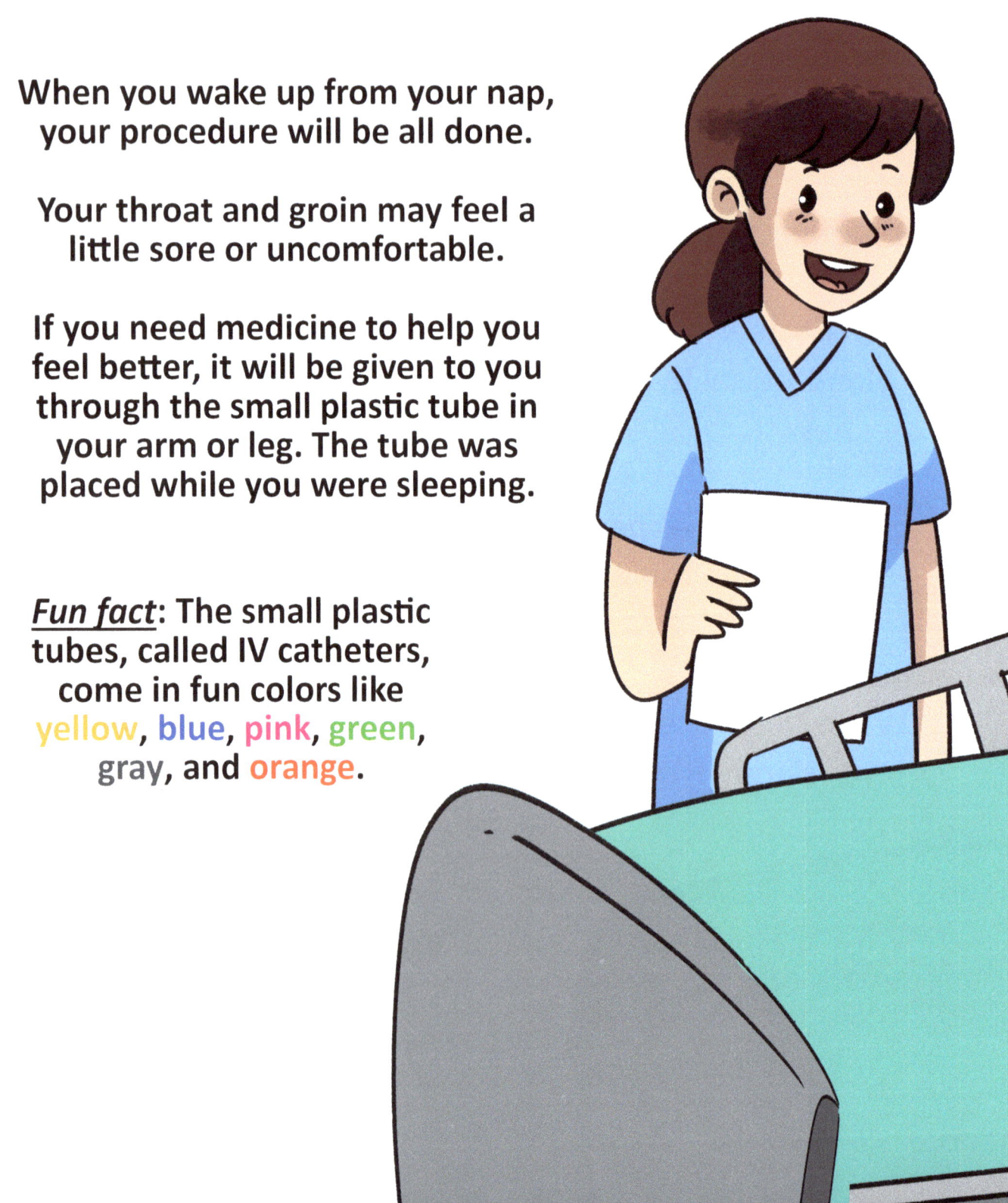

What color IV catheter will you get? Circle your IV color below.

yellow   blue   pink   green   gray   orange

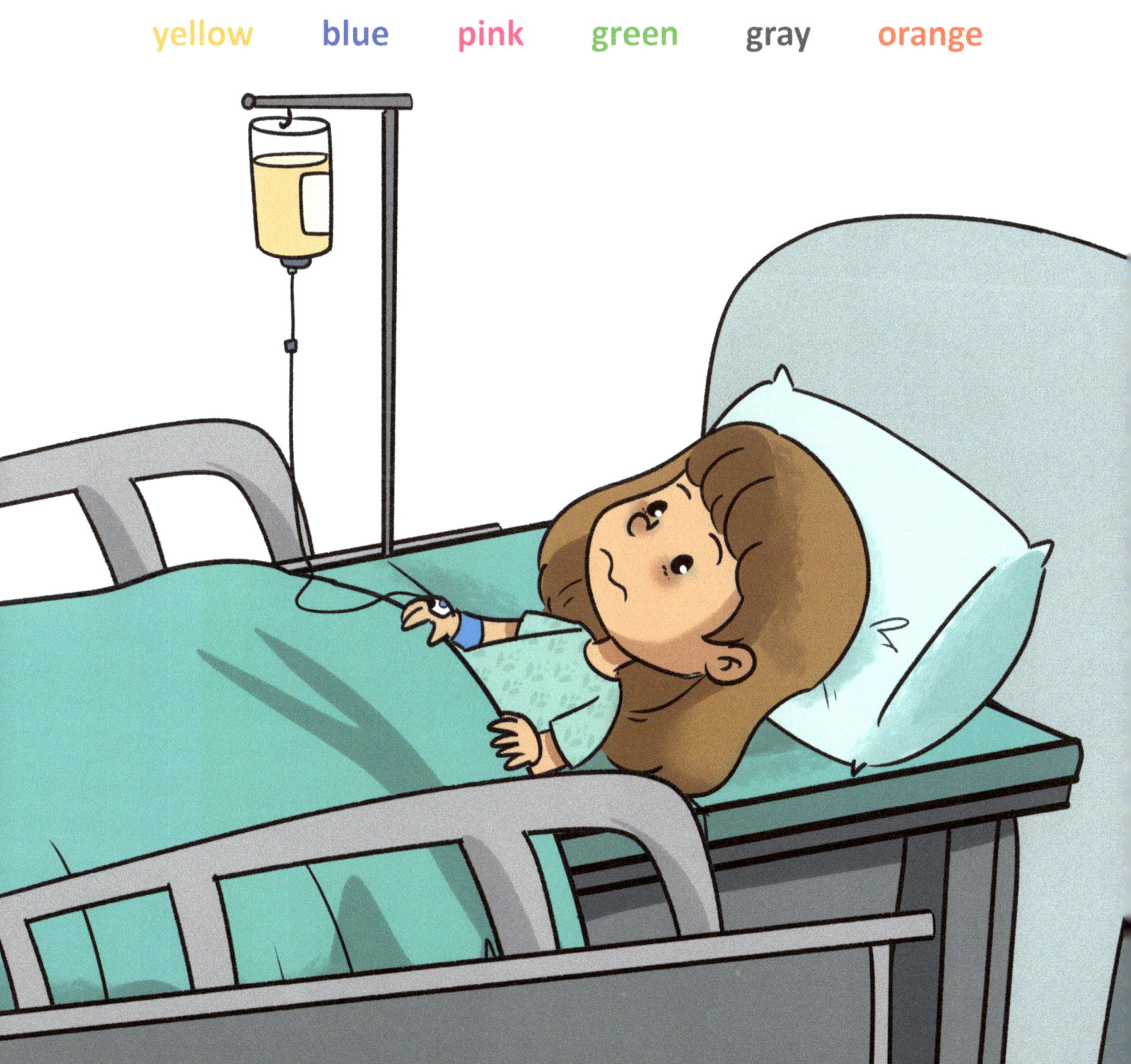

After your procedure, it is very important to lie flat in bed and keep your legs straight for some time. This helps your groin heal.

Sometimes, a board is used to help you keep your leg straight so your groin can heal.

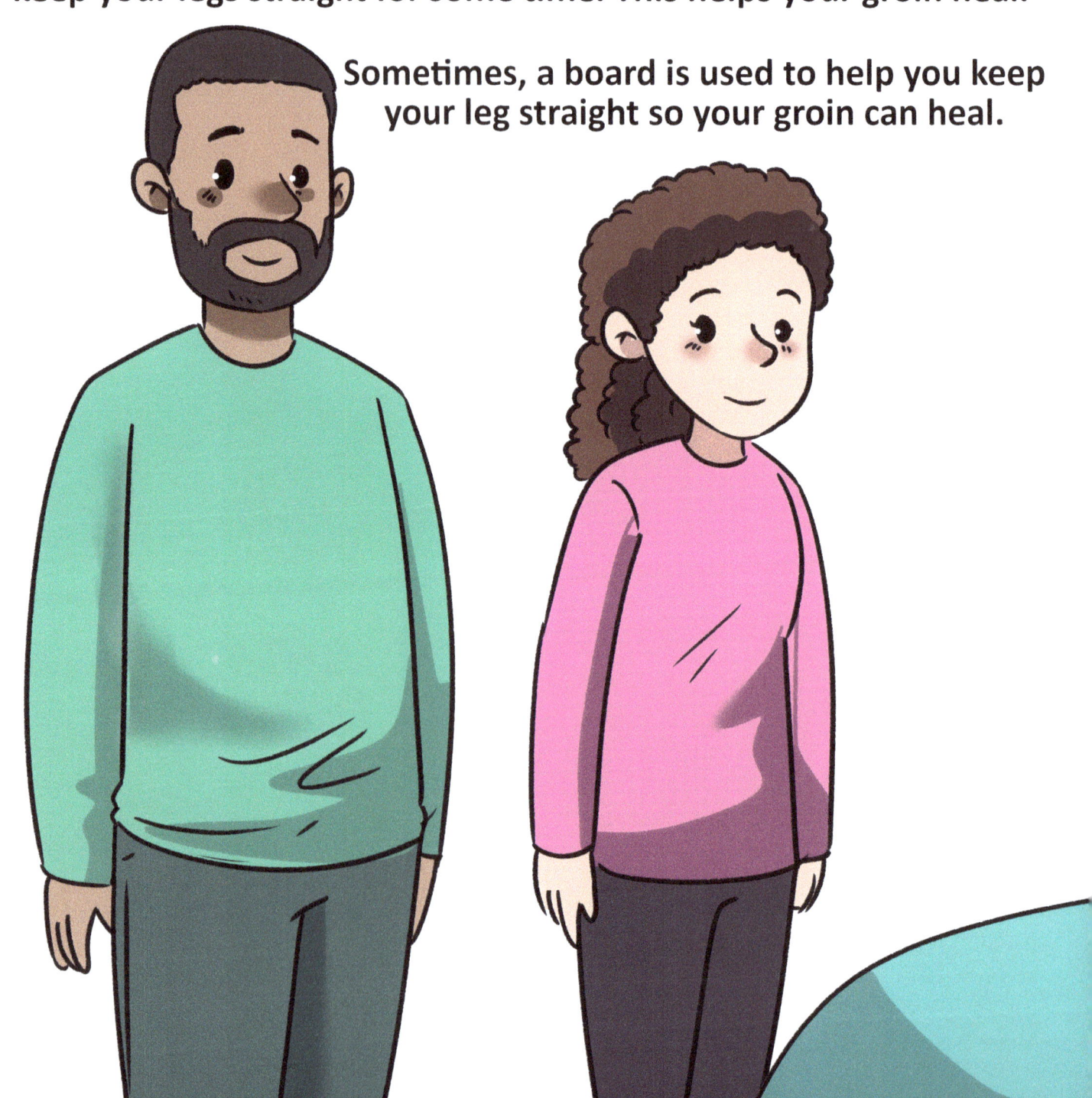

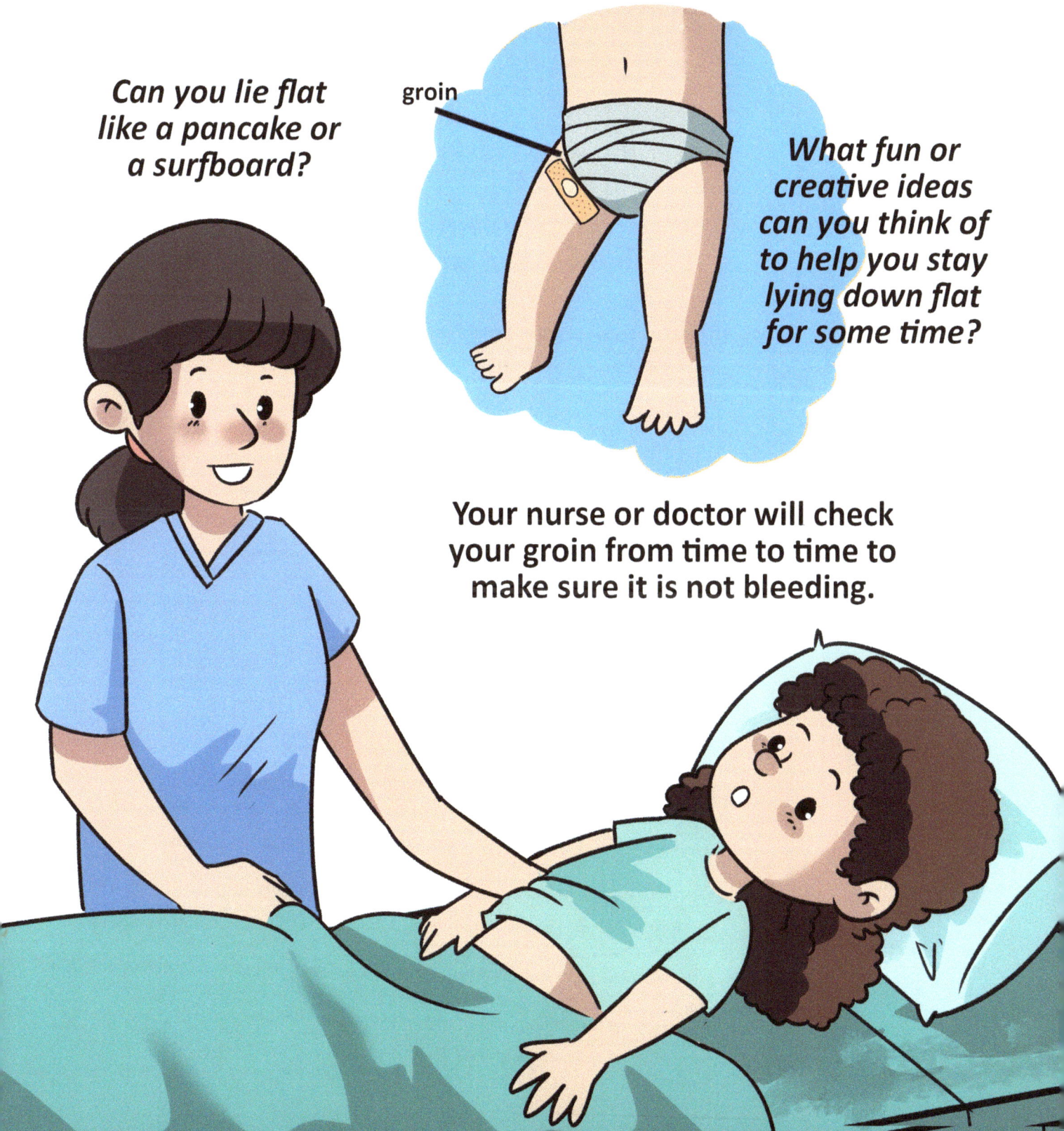

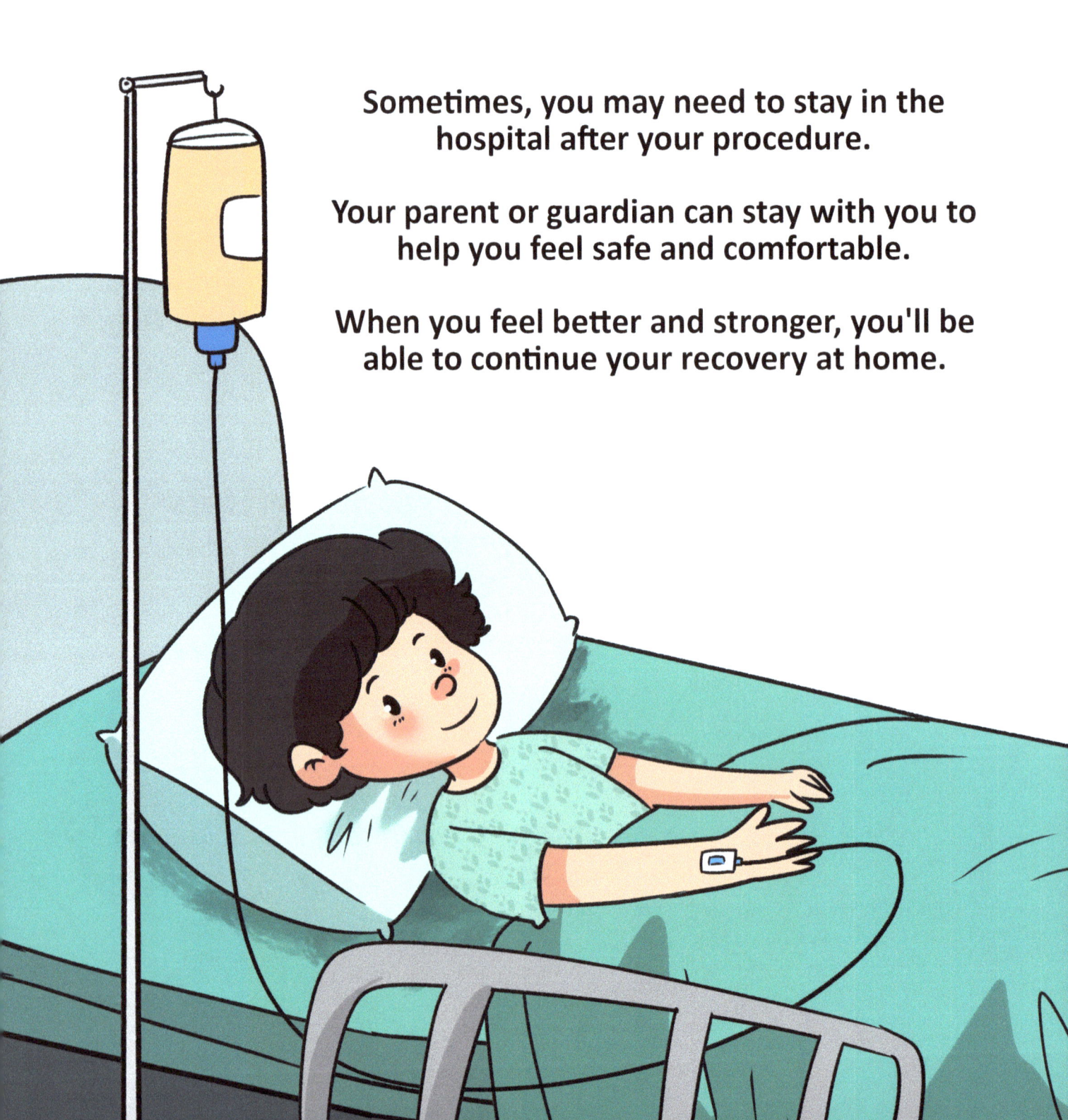

Sometimes, you may need to stay in the hospital after your procedure.

Your parent or guardian can stay with you to help you feel safe and comfortable.

When you feel better and stronger, you'll be able to continue your recovery at home.

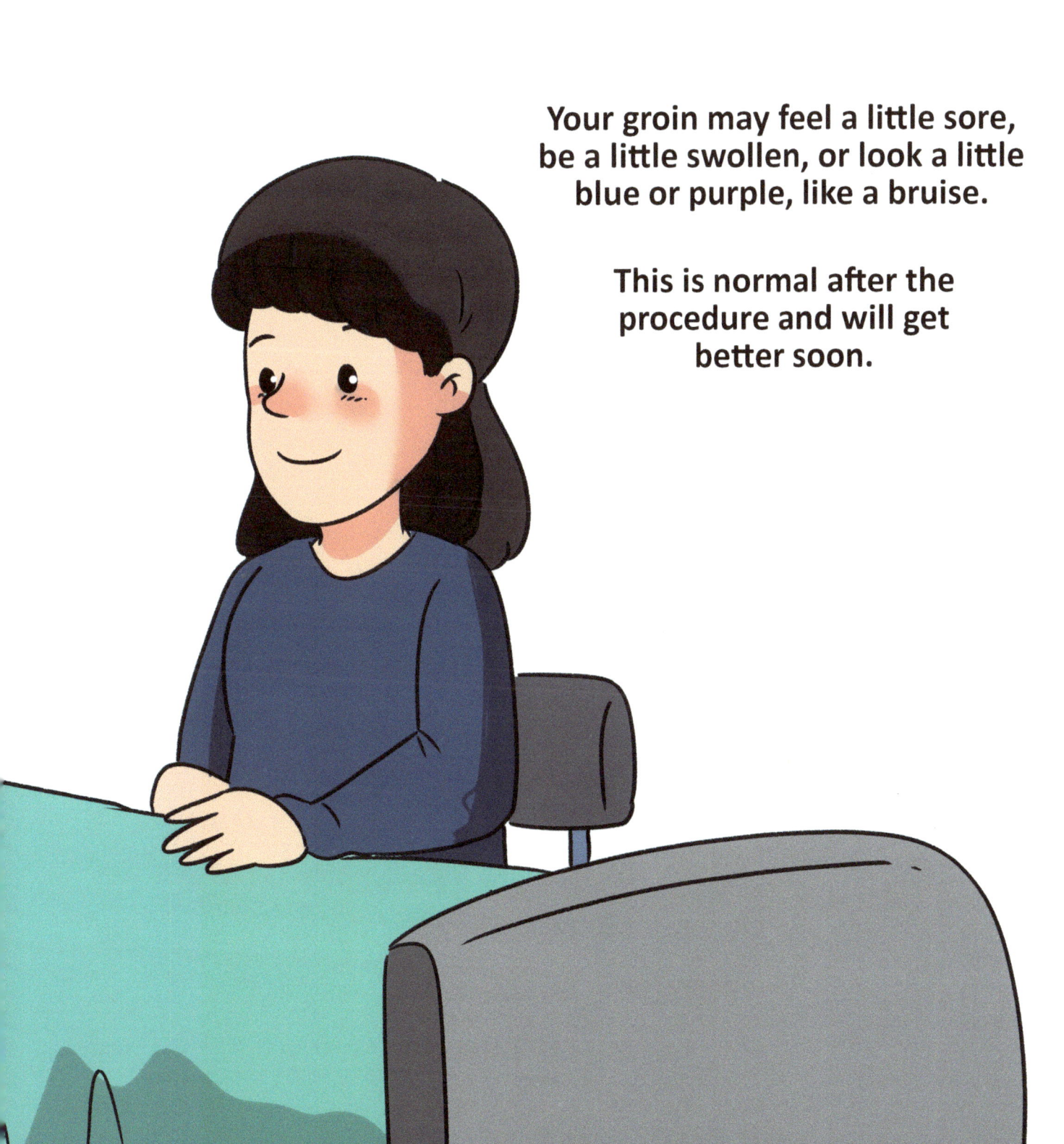

Your groin may feel a little sore, be a little swollen, or look a little blue or purple, like a bruise.

This is normal after the procedure and will get better soon.

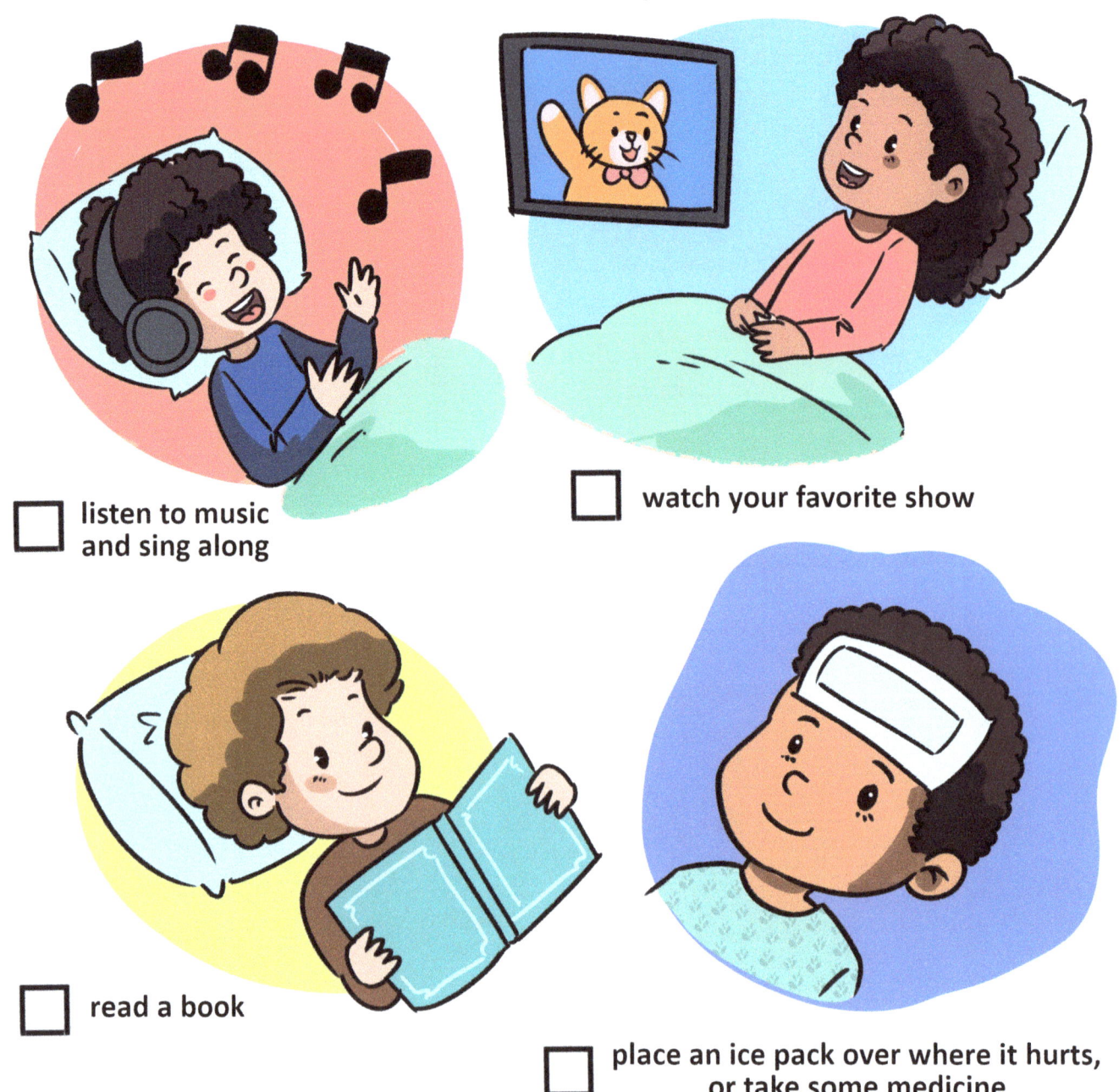

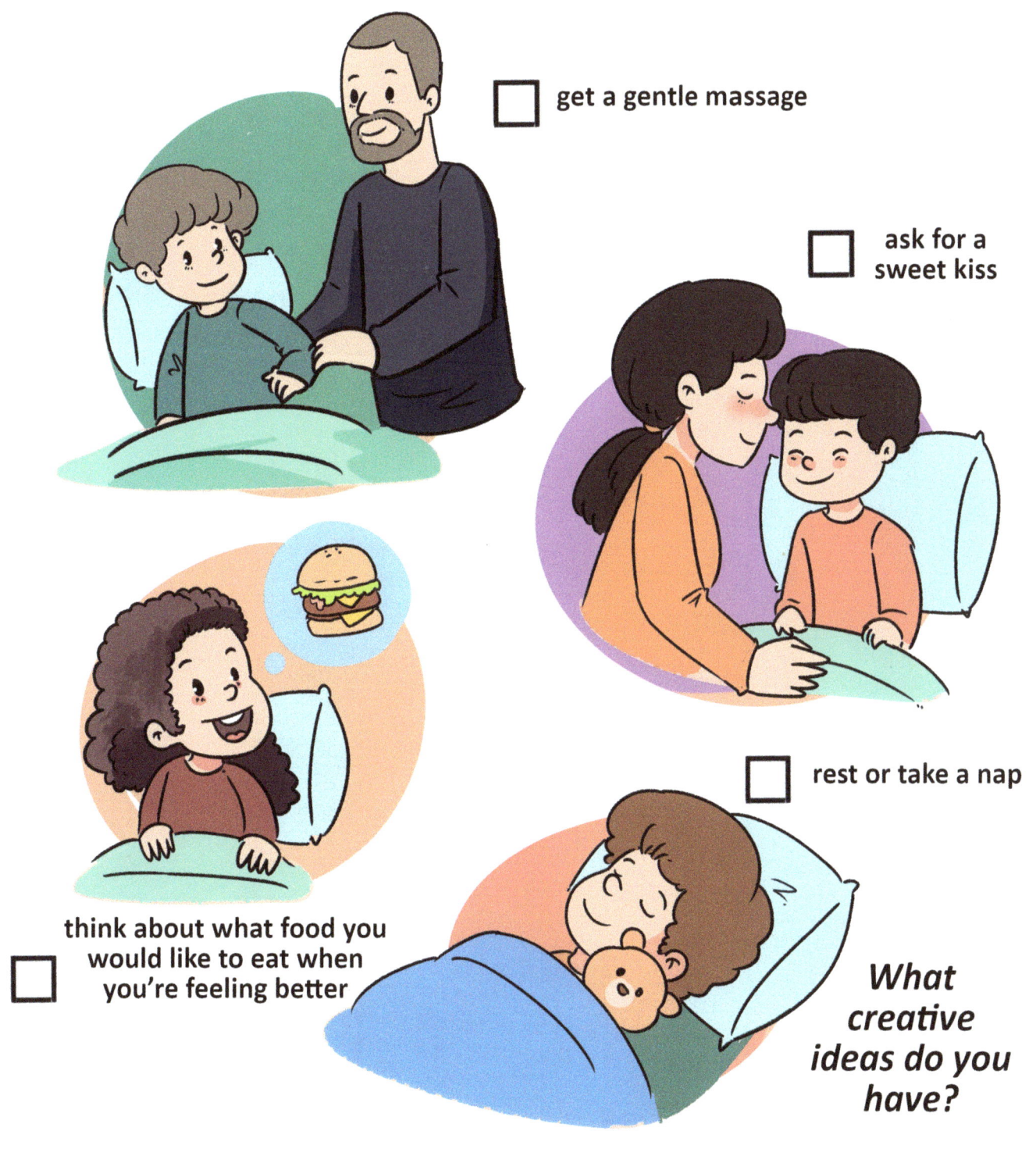

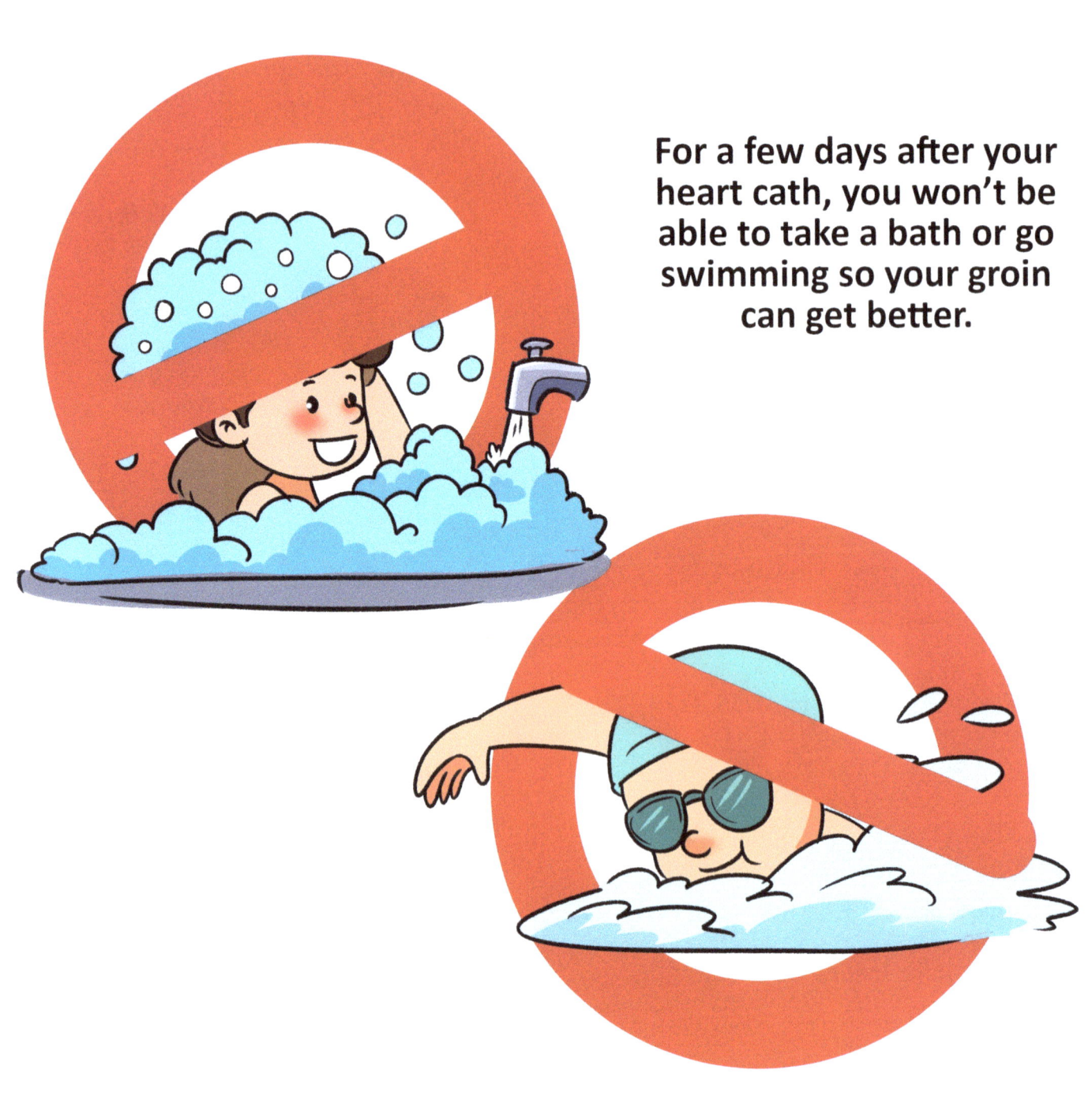

For a few days after your heart cath, you won't be able to take a bath or go swimming so your groin can get better.

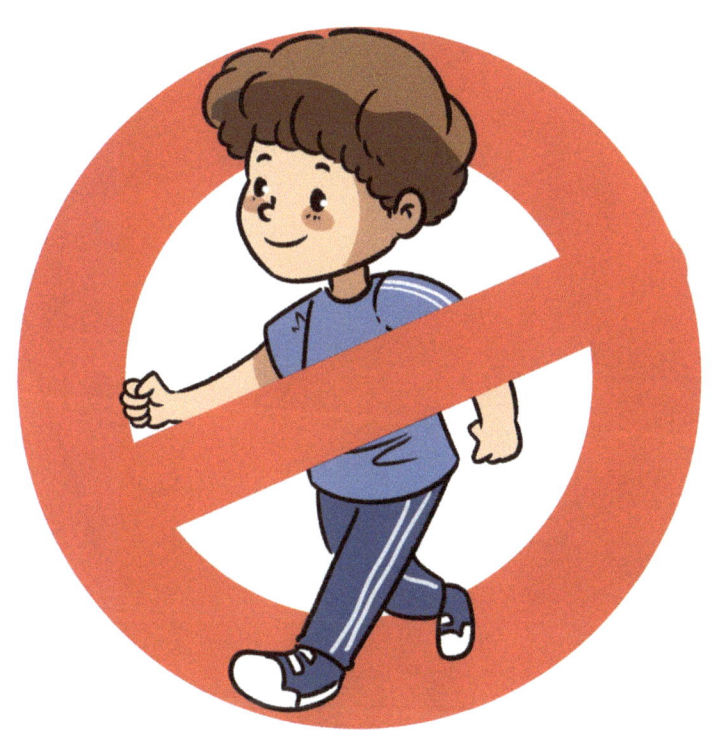

Don't worry, your doctor will tell your parent or guardian how to help keep your groin clean and dry.

Say NO to activities that could hurt your groin, like running or playing sports where you bump into others, for a couple of days.

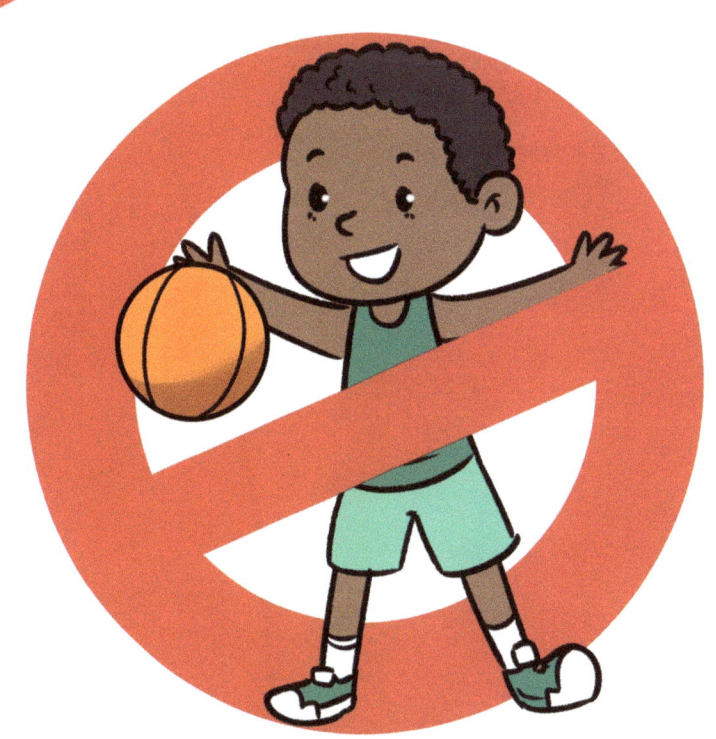

Soon, you will see your heart doctor to make sure you are healing well and getting stronger.

Your doctor will share ways to help you feel better, get strong, and stay healthy.

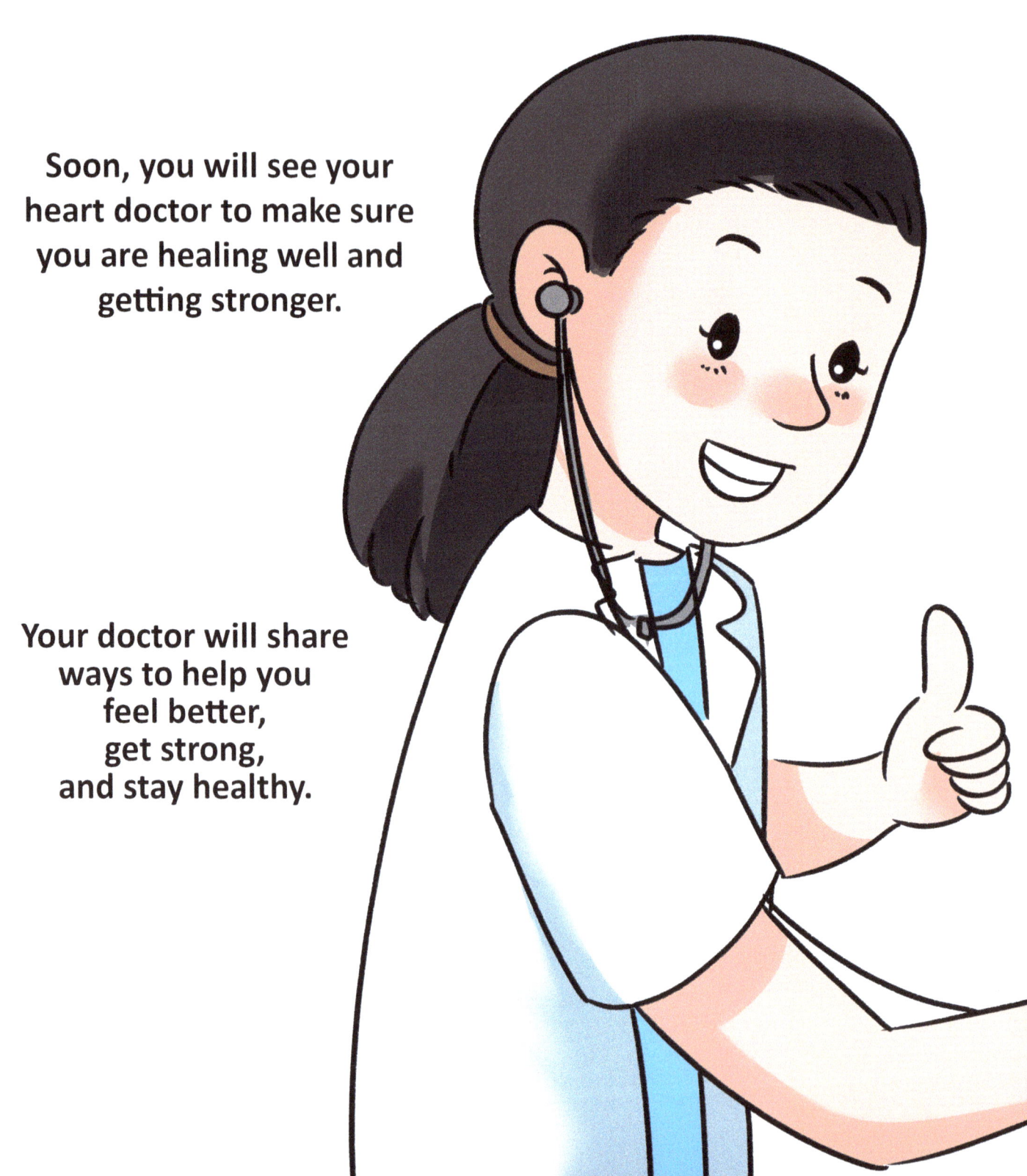

If you have any questions, your doctor is happy to help.

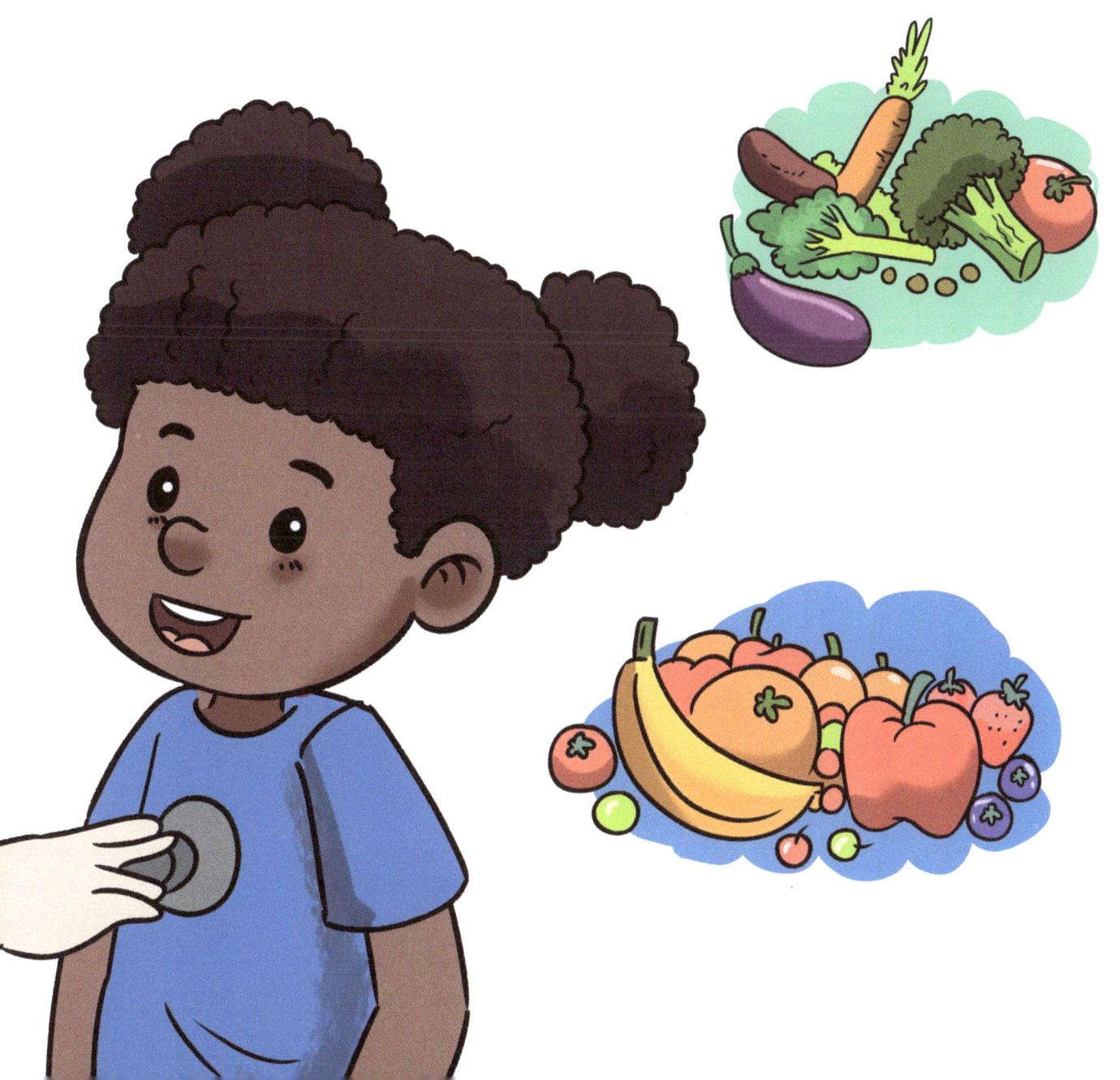

What will you do after your heart cath?

A party? A celebration?

What's your favorite way to celebrate?

Draw or write your party plan below.

Speedy recovery!

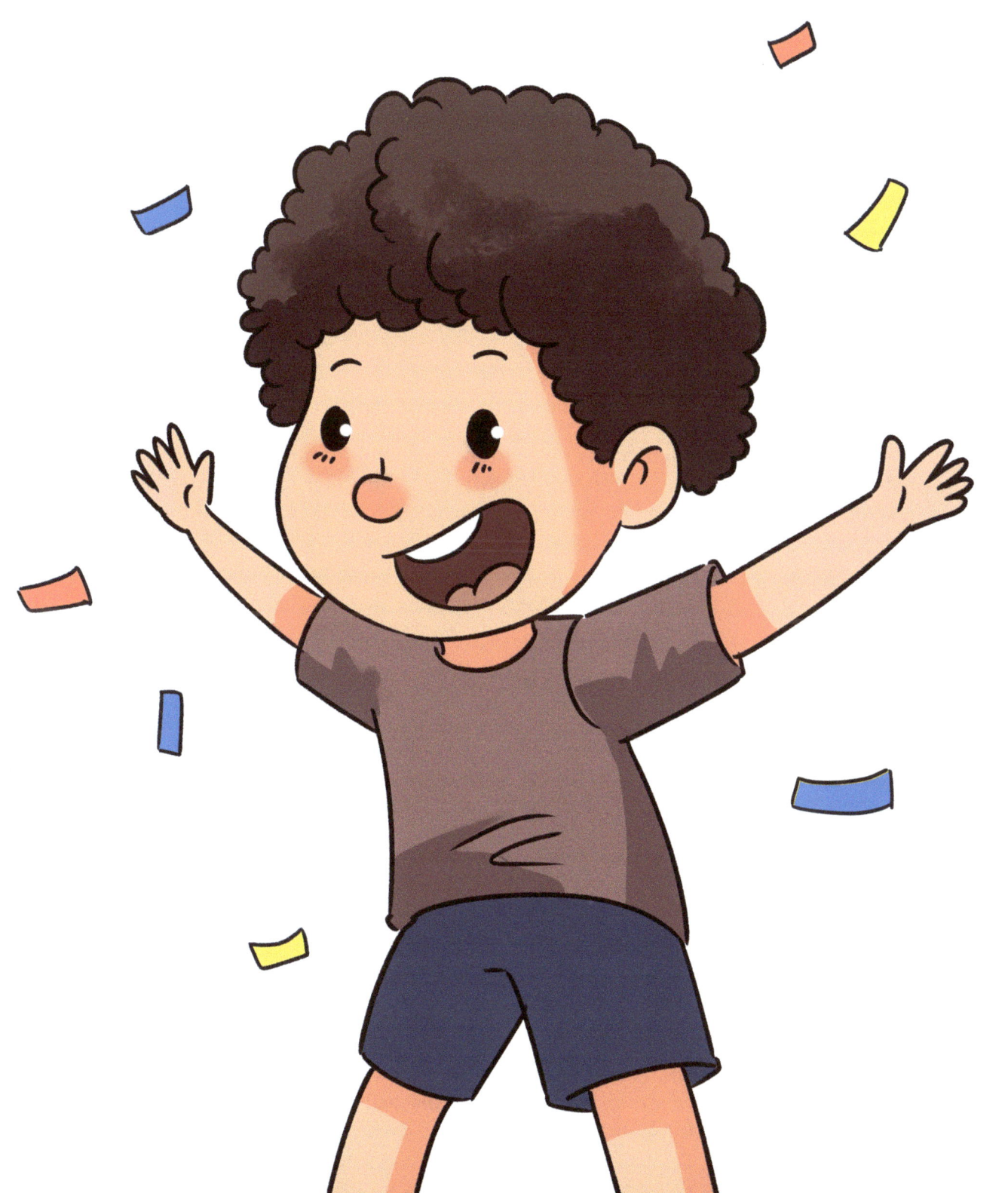

Notes for Parent/Guardian

- Placement of the intravenous (IV) catheter in this young age group is typically done *after* your child is asleep in the cath lab.

- After the surgery, it is common for children to feel confused, disoriented, or irritable, and they may cry, sob, kick, scream, or thrash around.
It normally takes about one hour for the anesthesia to wear off.

- If your little one enjoys daily baths, consider giving them a bath the night before the heart cath, as they may need to wait a few days after the procedure before bathing again. This is to help protect the wound site, keeping it clean, dry, and free from infection while it heals.

- Post-surgery instructions/restrictions:
Your child's doctor should give you specific instructions on (1) what your child can and cannot do during the recovery period, (2) the duration of the post-surgical restrictions, and (3) any post-surgical follow-ups. Additionally, (4) they should instruct what to watch out for and when it is necessary for you to bring your child back to the hospital in case of an emergency.
If they forget, please kindly remind them and obtain these instructions/restrictions before leaving the hospital.

Disclaimer

Please note that the illustrations are not drawn to scale.

This book is written for informational, educational, and personal growth purposes and should not be used as a substitute for medical advice.

Please consult your child's doctor if they need medical attention and to ensure the information in this book pertains to your child's medical condition and needs. I cannot guarantee what your child experiences is exactly what is being discussed in this book.

The author and the publisher are not responsible, either directly or indirectly, for any damages, monetary losses, or reparations due to information in this book. By reading this book, the readers agree not to hold the author and the publisher responsible for any losses as a result of any errors, inaccuracies, or omissions in this book.

Please keep in mind that your child's experience depends on the location, the facility, their medical condition, and the healthcare team.
Please use this book in conjunction with your child's doctor's advice. Thank you.

Did this picture book help your child in some way?
If so, I would love to hear about it!

www.amazon.com/gp/product-review/B0FG18PRXK

For other book titles, please visit:

www.fzwbooks.com

Connect with the author

email: books@fzwbooks.com
facebook/instagram: @FZWbooks

Books by the author

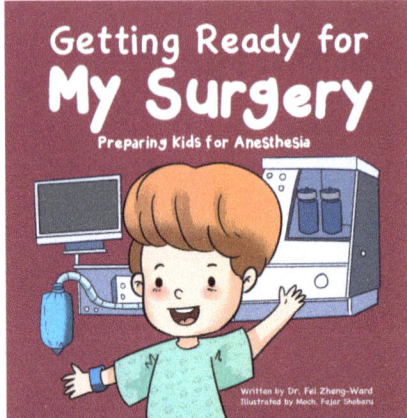
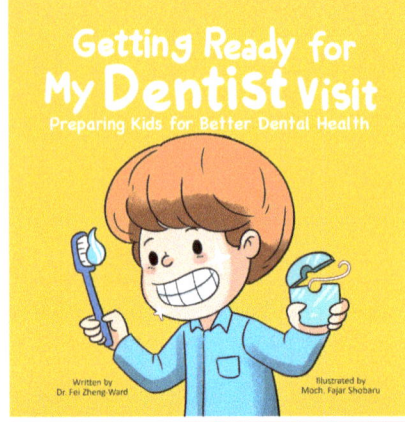
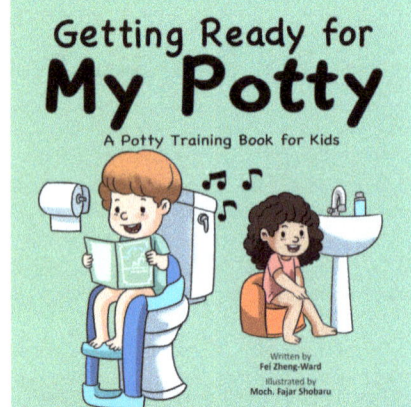
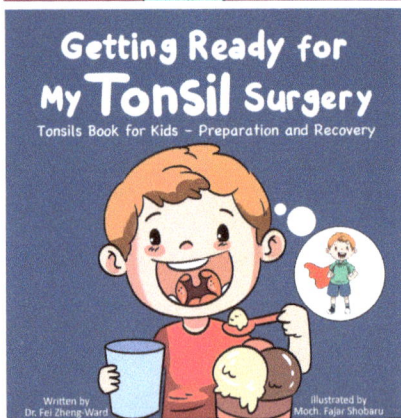
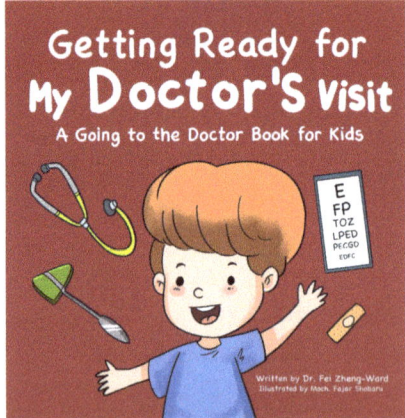
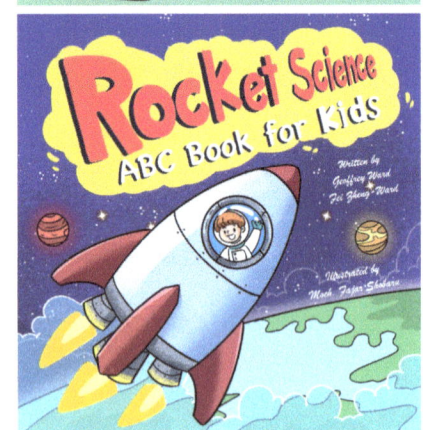
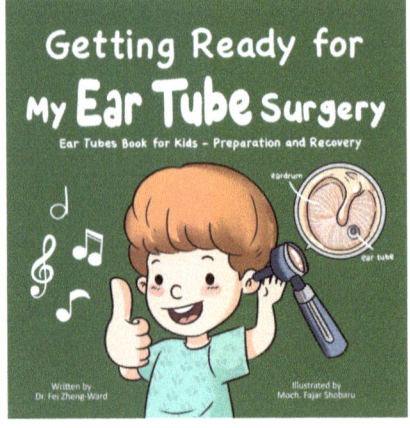
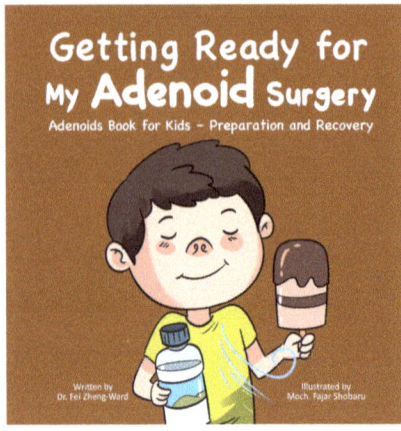
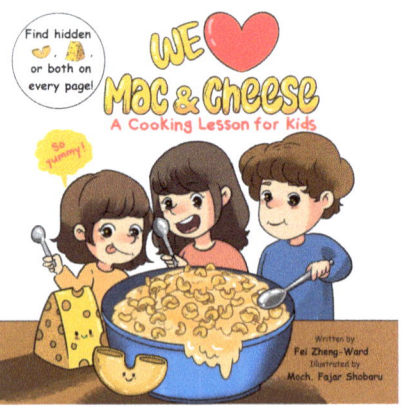

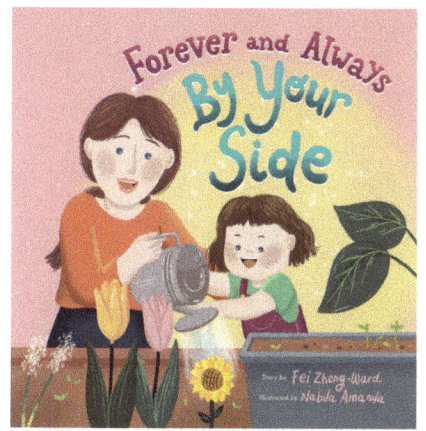
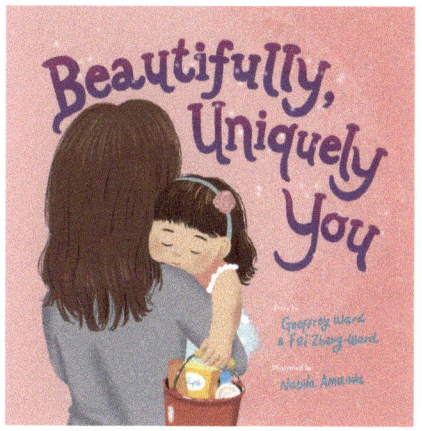
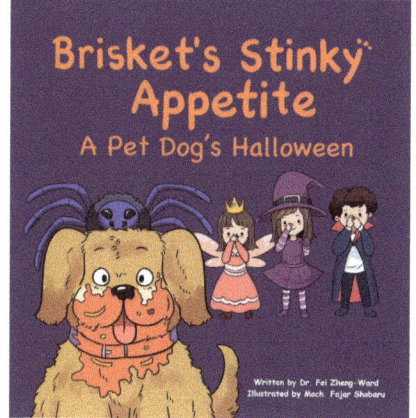
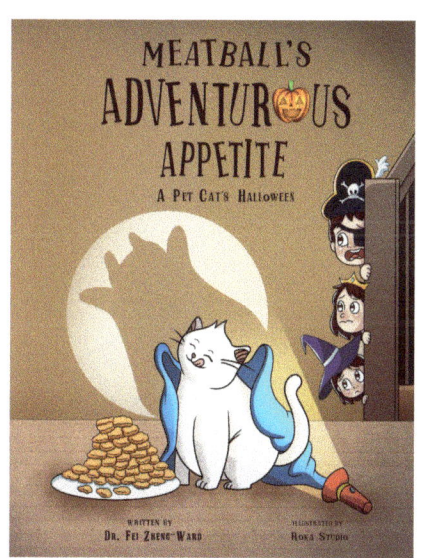
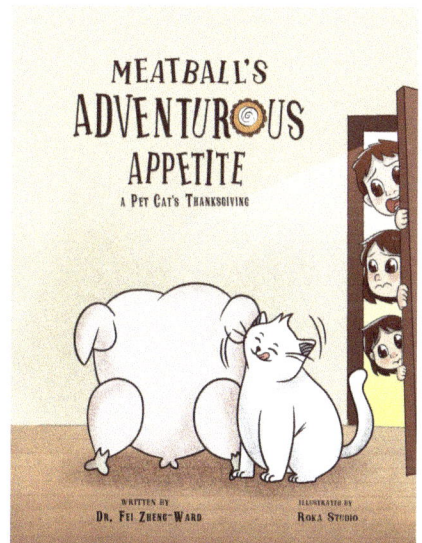
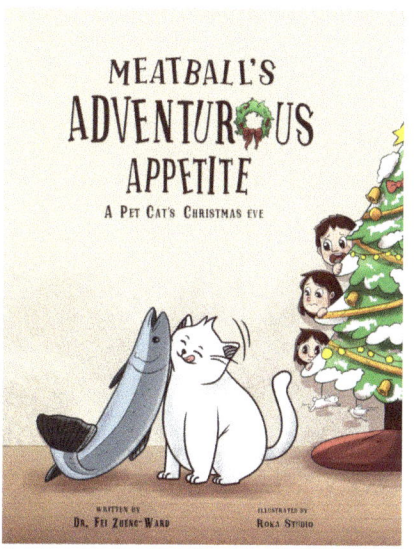
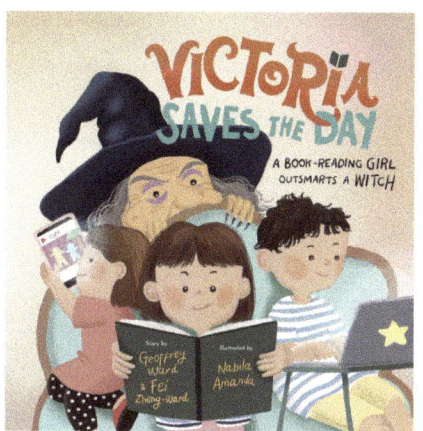
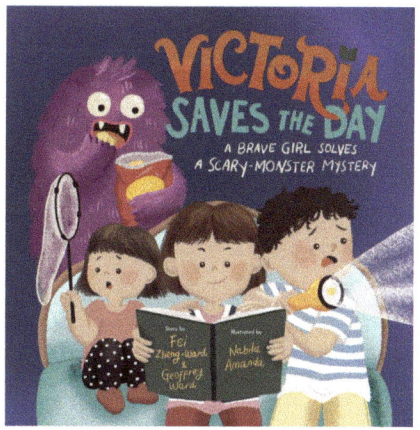
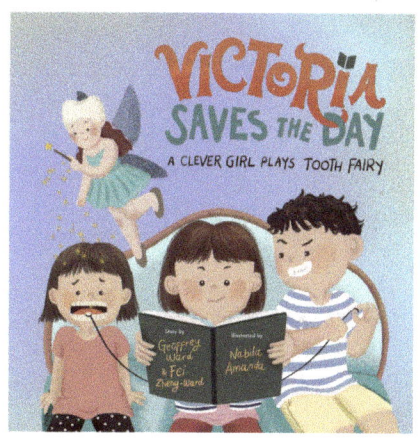

www.ingramcontent.com/pod-product-compliance
Lightning Source LLC
Chambersburg PA
CBHW042359030426
42337CB00032B/5162